FROM WITCHCRAFT
TO
WORLD HEALTH

by

S. LEFF, M.D., D.P.H.
Barrister–at–Law

and

VERA LEFF

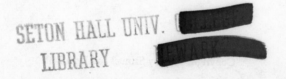

THE MACMILLAN COMPANY
NEW YORK
1958

CONTENTS

ACKNOWLEDGEMENT

Our thanks are due to the Wellcome Historical Medical Library for their assistance in choosing and in making available many of the illustrations in this book.

LIST OF ILLUSTRATIONS

INTRODUCTION

MAN'S QUEST FOR HEALTH

THIS book tells the story of man in his search for health. In recounting man's progress from witchcraft to world health, we must describe his first steps from the forest and jungle, and the eventful journey that has led to the concrete highways of the modern world; for in the struggle of man to live fully, the art and skill of medicine has been developed.

The history of medicine is more than a record of famous men and outstanding discoveries. It is the story of how men have lived and suffered, how they have struggled and triumphed; how they provided the conditions for men of genius to advance the campaign against ill-health—how mankind has made medicine.

In the early days even the most intelligent doctors could not explain the spread of infection, for there was no knowledge of germs nor any means of knowing; similarly, the skilful operations of modern surgery could not be performed until collective efforts had forged new metal and precision instruments.

This book is about the way men lived in different periods as well as about the illnesses from which they suffered, because these things are intimately connected; this can be seen even in a single industry where two men are employed in different jobs: the miner working underground is likely to contract silicosis, and the manager may suffer from diabetes or high blood pressure. When we look at the disease as part of the whole picture, and not merely alone, we are thinking along the lines of social medicine.

Medical students today are taught to adopt this broad and comprehensive approach to the science of medicine, and in their doing so, much that was flat and two-dimensional, printed words on a text-book page, suddenly springs to life; they see the patient in the round: a human being who has a family, a job, and a specific place in the community; and so the illness which the student wishes to understand and learn to treat is related to the human personality who is suffering from it and hoping for a cure. It makes medicine more

complex and more real; and therefore more promising, for success
in any sphere depends on how firmly we grasp the whole truth of
the situation we are trying to master.

As for the medical student, so for the layman, who shares with
our early ancestors a healthy concern for physical well-being. It is
fascinating to see how primitive man struggled to survive in a harsh
world, hampered by ignorance and lack of material resources. Now,
with an insight into social medicine, we can be more than merely
amused or interested by the quaint beliefs and methods of yesterday
(and even of today): we can begin to understand why and how
medicine progressed during countless generations. We can also understand how, as in the past, the story of medicine has been linked with
the story of mankind, so it will be in the future, with doctors and the
people together using the methods of social medicine so that all can
enjoy life and good health.

Chapter One

PRIMITIVE MAN

The Pattern Unfolds

THE story of medicine is the story of man: man's most constant problem has always been how to keep alive. Death is the final enemy, and to hold him off as long as possible man has to overcome famine and disease. Disease is as old as life itself, but by many victories civilised man has achieved an average life-span of three-score years and ten: a passage of time that is difficult to envisage in one sweep. How far, then, must we stretch our imagination to reach backwards five hundred thousand years, to try to understand how our earliest fathers battled with disease?

Prehistoric man survived in a world that was difficult and dangerous. How did he learn to defend himself, to protect his relatively weak body, and eventually to outstrip in power and achievement all other living things? To find the answers to these questions we must examine the relics that have been left, and try to clothe the bare bones with flesh and blood.

Thousands of generations and new races of man have come and gone, the vast majority without evolving even an elementary script, and so leaving no written records. Nevertheless, traces of their existence have been scattered about the earth, far apart in space and time; ready to give the answers to many of the questions man asks about himself.

From the remains of bones unearthed in Africa, Asia and Europe, we can get a picture of early man: the strong, hairy body so like an animal's, the low forehead and receding chin, the crouching posture ready for flight or attack.

In places as far apart as the river-valleys of France and the steppes of Siberia, evidence has been gathered of the ways he supplied his first needs from the raw materials available, even though no wooden implements have survived, and experts do not always agree about the stones which early man used as tools; some possibly having been

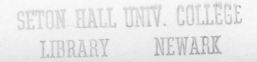

shaped by the action of wind and weather, but others clearly made by the deliberate hand of a craftsman.

About five hundred thousand years ago, man's ancestors emerged from their shelter in the trees of the thick forests to find their living in the green open spaces and river valleys. Like the prehistoric bear and lion, early man crept into the darkness of a deep cave to protect himself from the cold and the night. This was his first home; and like every home, it was left with the imprint of his daily customs. Students of man's history have entered such caves and have been able to reconstruct how the inhabitants ate, slept and worked.

Further knowledge can be gained from a study of primitive peoples who are alive today. The life of the Old Stone Age men is reflected by a few backward and isolated groups living in the jungles of Malaya and Central Africa, in the deserts of north-west Australia and South Africa, and in the Arctic regions.

The Beginning of Progress in the Stone Age

What gave man the ability to move far ahead of other animals, so that he overcame his fear and grew strong enough to master them?

His first advance was when he stood upright and freed his hands for more work. The fingers that scratched the earth for edible roots grew more sensitive, more exploring. Brain and hand working together in the endless search for food found that a suitable stone could be made to open a shell that had been too hard a nut to crack with the bare fist; a sharp stick in the hand was worth ten broken and bleeding finger-nails digging into the resistant soil for insect larvae and plants.

A stone in the hand of a man could kill a small animal, a squirrel or a rabbit; with stone spears and axes he could overcome more powerful beasts. But one man alone, even with a weapon, could not face an animal much larger than himself. So man, a rare creature on earth at first, lived and worked together in groups: he could be bold because he was united with his fellow-men.

Man's skill and inventiveness increased with his growing tasks, and his social organisation became more complex. It seemed a natural division that men should engage in hunting, and women remain nearer the settlement to care for the young. The women earned their living in a less strenuous way, which in time proved to be the most rewarding of all human activities, since part of their duties was to gather herbs and seeds, and they probably carried out the earliest cultivation of edible grasses and pulses.

Living and working so close to the earth, sleeping and rising in harmony with a natural rhythm, bound always for survival's sake to the closest observation of natural processes, mankind achieved at last a profound revolution: the Old Stone Age moved forward from a food-gathering to a food-producing economy; the era of the New Stone Age had begun.

As man prospered and his social organisation developed, he was able to produce a surplus of food to support specialist workers who improved their skill by devoting their whole time to their craft; in this way the witch-doctor emerged as a professional practitioner, receiving a share of the communal products in return for his services.

The Medical Problems of Primitive Man

The way in which man lived and struggled for an existence had a profound influence on the pattern of accidents and illnesses from which he suffered.

Violence struck at him from all sides: from the natural accidents of falling trees and rocks, from storm-blasts and shafts of lightning, from the savage beasts with whom he shared the jungles and the forests, and, most savage act of all, from hostile encounters with his fellow-men.

The earliest known case of a healed fracture is that of a reptile millions of years ago, and since then an increasing number of injured bones have lain scattered throughout the earth, testifying to the violent nature of the world wherein living things struggled to survive; and in the New Stone Age, the hand of man is clearly seen as an active agent in the general atmosphere of violence.

Man's brutality towards his fellows arose first out of the competition for land and out of rival interests of competing tribes. The skill that turned pieces of rock into useful tools was applied also to the creation of cruel weapons; the stone battle-axes and the flint daggers lying under glass in museums today are ancient witnesses to the murderous extremes to which man will resort when he lives in a harsh and unrelenting world.

The dark caves wet with moisture from underground rivulets and streams were the earliest form of shelter that men found in common with other animals. Such damp dwelling-places inflicted the age-old disease of rheumatism on the bones and joints of their inhabitants. Arthritic deformities can be seen in the skeletons of animals millions of years old, and so much evidence of rheumatism has been brought to light in the skeletons of prehistoric cave bears that it has been given the special name of "cave-gout". It is clear that the aching and creaking bones, the sharp spasms of pain, and the crippling deformities of rheumatic diseases tormented our ancestors as they do many modern victims of a damp environment.

With the absence of the remains of soft parts and with no written history of this time, it is difficult to detect the exact nature of the illnesses man suffered from. Infectious diseases must, however, have been prevalent; for although it is not possible to isolate specific germs, bacteria have been found in very early rocks, and microscopic examinations of coal have revealed various types of bacteria in the petrified remains of fish and reptiles. It must be assumed that they are the ancestors of present-day disease germs, and that germs are at least as old as man himself.

The type of food eaten by early man also influenced the diseases from which he suffered. Rickets, for example, has been found in prehistoric bones in northern countries where food must at times have been very scarce and sunlight rare. Famine must have stalked constantly behind and before him, periods of hunger alternating with those of glut.

Dental disease is an affliction not confined to civilisation; the experts agree that pyorrhoea and teeth discoloured with tartar have always been with us, even before the days of nicotine-staining tobacco. The teeth of primitive man show considerable wearing away, probably due to the coarse food he ate. Animals also suffered, but not to the same extent as man; according to the evidence available, there is no doubt that the pangs of toothache were felt in prehistoric times.

Magic and Medicine

It has not been easy to explore the world in which primitive man lived: it is even more difficult to see the world as he did. He has left some record of his inner vision in cave paintings and other works of art, and more can be learnt by studying the customs of present-day primitive societies. Significantly, primitive communities with a similar mode of living, yet far from each other in space and time, solve their medical problems in strikingly parallel ways. All primitive societies, ancient and modern, show the same trends of expression, whether it is in the art and skill of medicine, or in the traditions of their folklore.

Much of what happened to primitive man in his daily life mystified him; the diseases and physical disasters which took away his strength must have caused him fear and bewilderment. In his panic, he speculated feverishly about the cause of his afflictions, and he made serious efforts to overcome his powerful and unpredictable enemy, disease. Without knowledge of how his body was made and worked, primitive man had to face up to the attacks of germs and parasites, and the results of physical and mental disorders.

Like the animals, he had a natural defence in the instinctive quest for healing. The animal licks his wound; the primitive man seeks balm for his pain in the cool waters of a stream, or in the mineral springs and geysers which spurt from the earth close to his home. A four-legged creature hobbles on three legs, to rest the one that is injured; the man with the fractured limb creeps to his dark cave or hut. They both feel intuitively that rest is the great healer. A sick dog will seek the plants or grasses that can help to cure it; man may well have learnt from observing animals the medicinal value of herbs.

The inquiring mind always looks for a cause. Primitive man sought the cause of illness outside himself. Some things appeared connected, such as the falling rock which breaks the leg of the passer-by; where the cause was not obvious, it was always assumed that it must lie in some unknown outer force.

Other mysteries excited his fear and his imagination. Where was *he* when his body slept? What was the relation between these seeming brothers, sleep and death? Shakespeare re-echoed an age-long cry of wonder when he asked, through Hamlet: "For in that sleep of death, what dreams may come?"

Primitive man could well be afraid of his shadow, or identify it with his soul, for he did not possess, as every schoolboy does now, the simple scientific explanation. To modern man, dreams and nightmares can also be more vivid and fearful than reality; but we are not alarmed, because psychologists have given us reasons for their appearance. Primitive man could not say lightheartedly, "I ate something that upset my digestion and I had awful nightmares." To him the dreams were ghosts that singled him out for a weird visitation. It was logical to conclude, from the fear they inspired, that such spirits and demons could be malevolent, and by entering his body could cause pain and sickness.

Primitive man expressed his beliefs concerning the supernatural through his ritual and artistic practice.

As a hunter, his very existence had been bound up with the regular appearance of the mammoth and the bison on whose flesh he lived. On the stone walls of his cave he painted with black and bright yellow the living image of these animals; he drew them with all the skill and exact observation he had gained in the strict training of his daily life. When the very animals he had depicted appeared in the open for him to hunt, it seemed to him that he himself had brought this about by conjuring up their spirits on the walls of his home; if one form of magic was effective, why not others? So, with great fervour, primitive man performed his symbolic songs and dances, and made carvings on antlers and tusks; having thus stimulated and excited his own powers and determination, he went out to the hunt, better prepared to meet and overcome his prey.

But sometimes it happened that the hunt was unsuccessful, and some of his fellow-men were injured or even lost their lives. Then surely, it seemed to him, there must have been a change in the spirit of the life-giving animal: an evil demon must have taken possession. What could man do? As he had proved to himself that he could control the spirit, so he must overcome the demon and cast it out; but if it was too powerful, he could make efforts to appease it. So his magic rites and ritual became more involved, developing according to their own inner logic.

Early man encountered many setbacks in his daily struggle, but he also had his successes, and so it seemed to him that he could indeed influence the outside world by his ritual practices. This belief

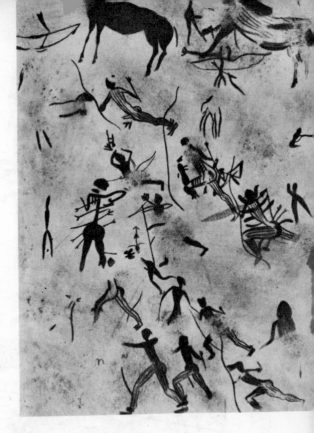

Spanish cave painting.

South African rock painting.

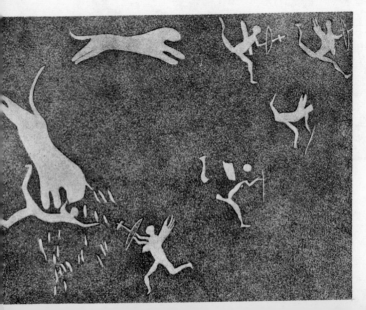

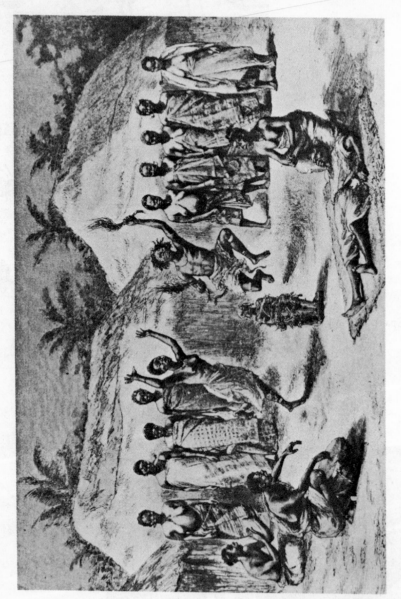

Consultation with medicine man.

persisted throughout succeeding generations, and ritual became a part of every activity, in particular of the treatment of disease.

Totem and Tabu

The twin pillars that upheld primitive tribal society were totem and tabu. As men lived and worked together in groups, they had to agree on common rules of law and order to protect the well-being and security of all. Since any major change from group customs could easily become a matter of life and death for the whole society, a strong emotional atmosphere surrounded the observance of these laws. The well-tried traditions were embodied in sanctified totems and strict tabus, and expressed with religious fervour in symbolic songs and dances. It was believed that ancestral spirits were the guardians of the tribal laws, and they were worshipped in fear and awe, for it was they who were outraged when tribal tabus were broken. In many parts of the world, even today, people go in terror of the "evil eye", which has the power to punish by sickness and death.

With this basic idea concerning the origin of disease, the main problem that occupied primitive man in seeking the causes of illnesses and accidents was why particular persons should have been singled out for affliction.

The way in which the disease actually was inflicted seemed obvious to him. He reasoned that as the trouble came from outside, something was added to the body by witchcraft and magic; evil spirits could do this, or certain people who had power over the supernatural. The strength of this belief can be seen today where in primitive races men have become ill or even died after being "pointed at" by an evil-wisher. The instrument used might be a hollow bamboo-cane filled with a dead man's bones, which is something real and terrifying in itself; or by suggestion the victim can be induced to believe that invisible arrows have been aimed at him. A common method of this black magic practice was to stick nails into a small effigy of the person it was desired to harm.

To the primitive men who believed that their society depended on the inviolability of the totem and tabu, someone falling ill or sustaining an injury was a stern warning that tradition had been infringed. How was man to deal with these supernatural forces that could so readily bring disaster not only to one, but to many? From earliest times he had struggled to master his environment by using his powers in ways that, to the modern man, can be explained in terms of psychology.

Primitive man joined battle with the spirits he feared. The strange and grotesque masks used in primitive medicine expressed a desire not only to frighten, but also to hide from the demons which bring ill-health. By similar reasoning, present day primitive peoples disguise themselves by colouring their skin, and by tattooing designs on their bodies as a special protection against disease.

They tried also to strengthen their bodies and constitutions against the onslaughts of the spirits. The totems of primitive societies were often symbols of animals from which the tribes were supposed to have descended. Because they wished so strongly to share the strength and agility of the totem-animal, members of the tribes dressed in the animals' skins and imitated in song and dance the habits and movements of the object of their worship. By similar logic, the characteristic movements of some diseases such as epilepsy inspired religious dances intended to appease the angry spirits.

The main aim of medical practice was to conjure up the spirits causing illness into the world of men, so that they might come under the spell of man's own magic-makers.

The Witch-doctor

From this non-rational approach, religion, medicine and magic became completely intertwined; and the specialist in the treatment of disease was something more than a healer: he was divinator, intermediary, appeaser, and sometimes avenger; and he frequently cured the patient.

What was he like, this witch-doctor? He walks the earth today, in the jungle clearings of Central Africa, and in other dark and remote parts of the world. He faces the demons of ill-health with a demoniac mask of his own creation; he frightens them with shrill rattle and booming drum; the very earth round the sick person shakes with the passion of naked feet stamping in a tribal dance in which he leads those who have been initiated into the art of medicine.

In his hand he carries his mysterious bag of tricks. This, too, is terrifying to see: the furry skin of a small animal stuffed full of herbs and potions, with the little head hanging downwards intact as it was at the moment of death—eyes staring, small jaws open to emit a last screech of fear. All this goes far to convince the patient that the evil spirits surely cannot long continue to defy the doctor's treatment.

The mind of primitive man is prepared for this mixture of suggestion and hypnosis by a lifetime of traditional training. People have always believed in the power of inanimate objects to give protection against disease or even to heal: the "rondelles" of bone cut from the trephined skulls of early men have served as amulets; shells, pieces of tree-bark, necklaces of animal teeth, balls of grease or dung have been treasured as healing agents.

Even in this scientific age, civilised people cling to irrational beliefs, such as in the power of lucky charms to ward off evil; many a motor-car, club and regiment has its mascot, whose damage or loss can cause an undue amount of misery.

In primitive medicine there is no clear division between magical and rational treatment. While both patient and doctor believe that it is an evil spirit that is being literally rubbed away, the aches and pains are in fact banished by expert massage. Many a child of the modern world has been soothed by mother "rubbing away the naughty pain". A powerful form of faith-healing is the transference of the illness to an inanimate object; the curiously carved dolls and statuettes which appear to us mere playthings are in fact an important part of the medicine-man's equipment, and they are of significant psychological value.

Problems of the Real World

The medicine-man, however, did not deal only in magic and ritual. He was, after all, engaged in a serious combat with natural phenomena, and by applying intelligent observation and skill, he arrived through experience at many practical ways of healing.

He related his study very closely to man's natural environment; he could read the signs of the weather and then direct the planting of crops; he understood how to control fire and water. From his generally superior wisdom he was credited with the power to predict the future and to diagnose illness from the study of the stars.

He may often have come to the right conclusions for the wrong reasons, but his medical skill can best be measured by the practical achievements of his work.

Besides his conjurer's outfit, the medicine-man had available a number of primitive but effective tools. Early neolithic saws of bone and stone were shaped to mimic the teeth of animals, the better to carry out their cutting and severing operations; the first probes and needles were adapted from fishes' teeth.

Once again the story of man's skill in healing can be read from the finds of prehistoric bones; from the way in which fractures healed, it is clear that human understanding was applied to the task of re-setting the injury so that the crippling effect of severe bone shortening was skilfully avoided.

The remarkable skull operation called "trephining" was frequently carried out in prehistoric times. Sharp flints were used to cut through skin and bone until a hole was made, and great skill was exercised to avoid injury to the brain; the wound was treated with herbs and natural oils.

Such serious operations were probably undertaken as a last resort in the treatment of diseases like epilepsy, where the behaviour of the patient in an attack, his losing consciousness, throwing his body about, uttering unearthly cries, would strongly suggest that he was possessed by an evil spirit. After the incantations and all the ritual of magic charms had failed, a final attempt was made, by cutting a small hole in the head, to let the demon escape. Trephining was probably used also for other ailments such as persistent headaches, lunacy and blindness.

Medicine men of present day tribes in East Africa, although having no knowledge of modern methods, conduct very skilful operations, such as protecting an open stomach wound with a piece of shell. Wounds are cauterised with heated spears, and thorns and fibre cords are frequently used to close them.

A very common treatment for all sorts of conditions was blood-letting. It was a matter of simple observation that a natural loss of blood, for example after a nose-bleed or after menstruation, resulted in a feeling of relief from discomfort. Linked with this was the belief that blood, in escaping from the body, also released the demons

causing the trouble. In Indonesia it is believed today that haemor-
rhages are caused by devils rushing from the body.

The usual method of blood-letting was to make a small wound
and then to suck the blood out through an animal's horn, but there
are examples of very small arrows which were shot at the forehead
of the patient, so that blood would run freely. Occasionally, many
superficial scratches were made in the skin to cause bleeding.

These were the main forms of treatment. The minor accidents
and ailments of everyday received the attention of the patient himself without recourse to the professional healer.

Primitive Medicine and Infection

For men to survive community life without serious infection certain simple precautions must be taken.

Primitive people learnt no doubt by long experience the need for
burying or burning refuse and human and animal excreta, and for
protecting water supplies from pollution. The dead were buried or
entombed, and burial places kept apart from the community. These
rational actions were inspired and maintained by primitive man's
belief in magic. He buried his excrement so that something which
had been a part of himself could not be worked upon by his enemies
and so indirectly cause him to suffer; he refrained from throwing
rubbish into the water because he did not want to offend the spirit
of the river; the elaborate ceremonial of the burial rites was intended
to propitiate the all-powerful ancestral spirits.

The tabus played an important part in the exercise of rules for
health and hygiene; for example, in regulating the disposal of refuse,
in segregating the sick, and in less rational laws such as that forbidding women during the menstrual period to go near flowering plants.

Although tribal customs arose mainly from superstition, many sensible methods of prevention have been handed down from generations past and are continued in present times by primitive peoples.

They believed that malevolent spirits could affect everything connected with the sick person: his clothes, his possessions, anything
he had touched; these fears led to measures which helped to avoid
infection. The sick were kept apart from the healthy, and many
communities were prepared to burn down the infected hut and its

contents; unhappily, in the case of some Indian tribes, with the ill person still inside. Other peoples who found themselves unable to cope with a spreading infection by the usual incantations and charms burnt the entire village and moved on to new land.

In the important disease, smallpox, there is evidence to show that many thousands of years ago a form of inoculation was practised by such widely separated peoples as the Hindus, the Persians, and the Chinese. Today, amongst the tribes of North and Central Africa, the operation is performed in the same way.

The medicine man makes a small wound in the arm of the person who seeks protection, and into the wound is rubbed some of the pus from an infected patient. This is done with the usual chorus of prayers and incantations, but it is clear that the practice has arisen out of rational observation; it must have been seen that a person who has survived smallpox is never infected again, and the intention is to give a mild attack deliberately, and so avoid a possibly fatal one.

The other side to this picture of intelligent medical practice is the grotesque smallpox cult associated with the priests of Shopono, the God of Smallpox. This cult still flourishes, and the priests terrorise the tribes and blackmail them for gifts, with the threat that by magic transference they can at any time inflict smallpox on a chosen victim.

An Estimate of Primitive Medicine

We have no reason to believe that primitive man's thinking powers were inferior to our own, but we know that he could progress no further than he did in the art and science of medicine, since most of his time and energy were taken up in the unceasing search for food and in protecting himself against the hazards of his environment; he had no tradition of science on which he could build his study, nor such aids as modern scientific instruments can provide to enlarge the scope of his own five senses.

He feared, and suffered from, many illnesses; and from his inability to explore the real causes, he created a tangled mass of superstitions, beliefs and theories which formed the basis of his medical practice; just as the child who fears the unexplored dark, peoples it in his imagination with terrifying things. We may smile at his ignorance and the fancies that misled him, but we should not forget that men at all times can feel and reason mistakenly about the things they do not really understand.

After all, primitive man used his crude instruments and social organisation to the full in his battle with nature and ill-health. Can more be said of the practice of medicine at other periods of history? Consider a child of modern civilised man, with the greatest endow-men of intelligence, reared in a remote jungle or village of Central Africa. Would he be able to practise medicine with any greater understanding and skill than that which was customary in his native surroundings?

Even today, beliefs which are held in common by a whole community, and sanctified by long tradition, are not easily questioned; and where the way of life has changed little over the centuries, there is small incentive to break through to new knowledge.

Nevertheless, without exact medical knowledge, man has survived all the dangers of a primitive existence. Within the limits imposed by his lack of information, he has used reason to help him make a clearing through the jungle of his world. He has struggled to control his environment, and all his intelligence and efforts have been directed to this end.

What Modern Medicine can give to Primitive Man

The connection between disease and malevolent spirits is so widespread amongst primitive peoples that no form of modern treatment can be successfully introduced unless consideration is given to deeply imbedded superstitions.

How important it is for modern administrators to understand and sympathise with the history of primitive peoples is well illustrated in the story of an attempt to provide drinking-water for a jungle village in Indonesia. The well was bored, but the population refused to drink the water. It was finally learnt that had the officials only consulted the village geomancer, they would have been advised to avoid boring the well into ground which might contain a vein of the dragon which sleeps under the soil of each village.

Clinics have been built for the benefit of backward peoples, and they have been shunned because the doors opened in the direction from which evil spirits come, or the screen which keeps them out

has not been put up; or the buildings have perhaps been erected in
a ... which was once a burial-ground.

...e are many ritual ceremonies connected with child-birth which
...ore to the mother than does the hygienic medical treatment
...vilised maternity ward. Some African tribes place the baby
on the naked earth as soon as it is born, so that it may absorb from
the soil the spiritual force of its ancestors; naturally there is a strong
prejudice against entering a maternity hospital where such an important traditional act is impossible. A simple compromise could be
made by permitting a handful of the soil from the village to be
brought to the mother so that the new-born baby can be touched
with it. Primitive peoples are not the only ones who attach a symbolic
significance to the land of their fathers.

Hospitals which forbid the wearing of amulets and charms believed
essential to keeping off evil spirits, are undermining their own efforts
to bring the benefits of modern medicine to primitive people.

A common obstacle to treatment is raised when the modern doctor
ignores the profound significance which the primitive man attaches
to blood. To give up a drop for medical examination means that a
vital part of himself has passed into unknown hands, and through it
any harmful spell could be laid upon his body, his will, or his future.
It was found in Afghanistan, during a mass campaign against syphilis,
that in order to convince the mountain-dwellers that their blood was
not to be used for some magical purpose, the laboratory had to be
conveyed by mule to the people so that they could see for themselves how the samples of blood were used for diagnosis.

With patience and understanding, all such difficulties can be overcome.

What Primitive Man has given to Modern Medicine

The early mothers of the race who patiently gathered wild flowers
and herbs and distilled their essence into pain-relievers, stimulants,
laxatives and sleep-inducers, were gathering gifts for the sons and
daughters of all time.

Today we use opium, coca, ephedrine, cascara sagrada, digitalis,
ipecacuanha, and many other drugs whose names breathe of the
remote past and distant lands; and our extended knowledge and

experience will be passed on to the enrichment of later generations.

Since earliest times the interaction of mind and body has occupied the attention of the healer, and in the poetic frenzy of the witch-doctor, the faith of the Christian Scientists, and the scientific treatment by hypnosis of the modern neurotic, there is a connecting thread of intuition and understanding.

In modern times warts *do* disappear by suggestion; rheumatic pains do respond to red flannel; and here it must be noted that it is the colour, not the material, that has the hypnotic significance; just as it had when primitive man first defended his door against evil with a red-painted figure.

We recognise that our understanding of disease cannot go far beyond the limits of our accumulated experience. Primitive man did the difficult pioneering which has enabled mankind to make progress, sometimes gradually, sometimes in a great surge forward, in the advance towards good health.

Chapter Two

EGYPTIAN MEDICINE

Mankind takes Roots

ABOUT five thousand years ago, great changes occurred in man's way of living.

Over thousands of years the world had gradually become more habitable for man; climatic changes had turned frozen wastes and desert areas into fruitful lands fertilised by rivers teeming with fish.

Communities were drawn towards the rivers, where they settled down to a pastoral life with the added advantage of convenient transport along the river highway. The clear night skies revealed to men's watching eyes a pattern of stars which guided the navigator and helped the husbandman to plan his seasonal tasks.

As they settled down in these favourable circumstances, man unearthed a new source of riches—copper and tin. The flame which had mastered other stubborn elements now helped to produce bronze, and the communities who were first to exploit the new element soon won victories with their more effective arms over those who wielded the old stone weapons.

The spoils of victory included thousands of captives, who became the property of the section of the community that was accumulating land and bronze, and creating a monopoly for themselves and their heirs. The captives were more valuable alive than dead, for they were set to work with the new, more adaptable and hard-wearing tools, and by their unceasing labour the general wealth was vastly increased.

So men began to develop highly complex civilisations concentrated on the great rivers of the world; along the Nile, where the Egyptian Empires ruled for over a thousand years; the Euphrates and the Tigris, which nourished Assyria and Babylonia; the Indus, which was India's "river of life"; and the Yellow River, the great waterway of China.

The achievements of these different nations varied; for example, the Babylonians were ahead in their knowledge of astronomy and in formulating a medical code; India was more advanced in surgery, and China in organising a system of State Medicine.

The Story of the Tombs and the Written Word

Egypt, with her almost intact tombs and many written records, has bequeathed to humanity a fascinating picture of the life and culture of a bronze-age civilisation, and it is to Ancient Egypt that we must go for the story of man's search for health when first he became a maker of cities and empires.

The excavations of the past hundred years have revealed an astonishing variety of goods which tell in their own way of the everyday life, hopes and fears, the religious, medical, and scientific ideas of the Egyptian citizens who lived thousands of years before the Christian era.

One of their great achievements, not only for the Egyptians but also for future historians, was the use of papyrus, to which our modern paper is related. On this flexible and easily handled medium, made from strips of a weed which grew extensively along the Nile, the Egyptians were able to record their story. Legal contracts dealing with property in land and slaves, historical events, love poems, medical tracts and magical potions, geometrical measurements and prayers for the dead: life had become so intricate that means had to be invented to aid the memory and help men in their dealings with each other.

The Babylonian method of writing by chiselling signs on stone was a rigid form of communication; the Egyptian papyrus gave freedom to man's recording hand, and thanks to a suitable climate, tens of thousands of papyri have been preserved to this day. Many have been taken from the tombs where they were placed to protect the mummies from evil; because of the Egyptian's intense preoccupation with the fate of the dead, we have been able to gain a vivid picture of the living: and so these people have found immortality in a way they little dreamed of.

In spite of the direct evidence we have of the tools the Egyptians used, their instruments and weapons, and their written records, caution must be shown in drawing conclusions about their civilisation; we cannot say we are in possession of all the significant facts. Until

the discovery at the end of the nineteenth century of the Edwin
Smith Papyrus describing surgical techniques, we knew only of a
mass of magico-religious formulas which showed no marked evidence
of medical knowledge.

The Life of the People

It is evident that the pastoral economy of peoples like the Egyptians
developed to a high degree, drawing its strength from the labour of
large numbers of slaves and qualified technicians.

Within the framework of this advanced economy, with the Royal
House commanding every luxury at the centre, the great cities of
Egypt were built; cities which were graced by impressive temples
and mansions, and shamed by rows of squalid back-to-back work-
men's huts; cities which were hives of industry and models of organisation, but where the toiling people were driven on mercilessly by
the whip of the overseer.

It was not uncommon for the houses of the masters to contain as
many as seventy rooms, with bathrooms and often a courtyard, a
garden and a pond; they also had their country retreats where they
could pass their leisurely hours in sport and entertainment; the majority of the people had no escape from their narrow streets where
they lived, deprived of fresh air and space.

As the country was fertile, there was generally a good supply of
food; in times of drought it was, naturally, the slaves who felt the
resulting shortage. The usual diet included bread, fish, and the meat
and milk of domesticated animals, together with fruit, vegetables and
various cereals. A good basic daily ration was considered to be three
or four loaves and two jars of beer. The bread of the people was
coarse and hard on the teeth; fish prepared in a variety of ways was
a popular addition, and sometimes it was eaten raw, sometimes dried
or pickled. The fruit and vegetable markets could make a fine show
with heaps of melons, cucumbers, olives, dates, figs, grapes, onions,
leeks and garlic.

The people dressed simply, usually in one-piece tunics made of
white linen. The hot weather made extra clothing unnecessary, and
children often ran about naked. Cleanliness and physical fitness were
encouraged by these sensible customs.

As in many Eastern countries today, child marriages were the rule, and the young girl dedicating her toys and playthings to the Gods immediately took on adult responsibilities. Mothers bore many children, but the infant death rate was very high. Most men had only one wife, although legally they could take into the household as many concubines as they could maintain, and the wealthy took full advantage of their privileged position; Egyptian customs helped to produce prostitution, which was accepted as a convenient institution.

As the Old Testament relates, the working conditions of Ancient Egypt were notorious for extracting labour from slaves and peasants. The people toiled incessantly at all the essential works: canals, dams and water basins for flood control were always under construction or repair; agriculture also claimed many hands. To be sent to work in the mines was a death sentence.

Ancient Egypt could be proud of her fine craftsmen, but their position was that of serfs; they worked for nothing more than their food. The ruling class developed tastes which used all the time and skill of these craftsmen. Glaziers, jewellers, seal-cutters and potters were employed in fashioning works of art for the enjoyment of their masters and the glorification of their dead. The secrets of the craft were often passed from father to son; a knowledge of the appropriate incantations was considered as important as good workmanship.

In this increasingly complex society many new problems arose, which could be solved only by using rational scientific methods. Calculations had to be made of how much seed was needed for sowing and how fruitful the harvest was likely to be; a calendar to help navigation had to be based on astronomical studies and reckonings; the science of geometry was evolved to help in the surveying of large buildings, granaries, tombs, canals, dykes and other ambitious projects; rough weights and measures had to be standardised, as primitive forms of exchange gave way to the introduction of money as a common symbol of value.

So there arose from the people priests, astronomers, architects, physicians and administrators; a class which found it essential to evolve a special tool, a written language, which they refined and polished in the course of their work.

The exchange of experience and knowledge gained in dealing with these difficult problems helped all the intellectuals to develop a rational approach to their work. The necessity for prayers and incantations was not questioned, but it was recognised that, however potent the magic charms buried in the foundations of a new building, the construction would fail if the calculations and engineering were at fault.

A serious weakness in the work of this group was that the clerks, priests and physicians were not much concerned with the problems and sufferings of the multitude; their interests were linked to the requirements of their patrons, the small but powerful class in whose hands all the surplus production was accumulating.

Witchcraft and Religion

The magic and mysticism which previously had dominated man's view of the world became transformed in the Egyptian era into a strict religious dogma which served a useful purpose in maintaining the State under a unified central government.

Pharaoh, the King of Kings and of the lesser landowners and nobles, was also the supreme God whom all Egyptians must serve. This was the opposite to the belief of the primitive clan whose religion dictated that all must work together for the common good. It was, however, imposed upon the slaves and peasants with an overwhelming show of power, and in their obedient toil they made the base upon which the system rested.

So closely was man's destiny linked with the goodwill of the gods, that the people, illiterate and ignorant, felt helplessly dependent on the priests and physicians; they were taught to believe that these men were their only protectors against an evil fate.

As there was general ignorance about the cause of illness and death, it was easy to substitute for rational thought the belief that any attempt at revolt against enforced drudgery would be punished by the gods with all the sickness people dreaded. In exchange for tribute, Pharaoh, his priests and physicians promised protection; they alone had the monopoly of learning and knew the secrets of the medical lore that had been handed down on the sacred papyrus. Into these all-powerful hands the people delivered the most part of the fruit of their labour. On special feast days, priests distributed food from the temples and led the people in religious rites and dancing. Thus inspired, the masses returned to their work duly grateful for the generosity of their rulers.

The study of the stars which had proved so helpful to the science of navigation was intermingled with the lore of astrology, which was pure magic. The changes in the heavens with eclipses, comets and equinoxes were believed to foretell great events, wars, famine and epidemics; the position of the stars at the moment of a man's birth determined his character and his future. The priests alone could find and interpret the omens, and in Babylonia tall towers were built to help their inspection of the skies. In addition, unusual signs were sought for and interpreted; any rare event, such as an abnormal birth amongst humans and animals, was taken to be a warning of disaster.

One of the dominating passions of the Royal Household of Egypt and its retinue was to ensure a happy and prosperous after-life, no doubt because they were so comfortable and well-cared for in this life that they wished to perpetuate its joys for ever. The priest-physician, who applied his thought and skill to their well-being and paid close attention to their particular ailments, employed much ingenuity in creating spells and incantations to protect the dead from the evils that might haunt their tombs.

Just as the Sphinx and the Pyramid dominated the Egyptian land-scape, the doctrine of life-after-death governed the hopes and fears of the Egyptian people. A vast amount of energy was spent in the ritual surrounding mummification; even those whose life on earth was one of toil eased only by a few simple pleasures yearned for im-mortality. Charms and amulets were buried with the dead: gold, lapis lazuli and precious stones for the wealthy; linen amulets and small bronze ornaments for the poor and humble.

For their important patrons the priest-physicians composed a Book of the Dead, and into it they poured all they had learnt of the magic ways to protect men from the evil eye.

In accordance with the wish to surround the dead person with all he had treasured, the embalmers mummified the creatures that had been pets or companions, including cats, dogs and even a mouse and a honey-bee, complete with sarcophagus in the shape of a small hive. The craft of embalming the dead improved until it reached a fine art, and it is due to this skill that it is possible with the help of modern equipment, including X-rays, to learn much about people who died thousands of years ago.

The Egyptians made a positive contribution to medical science by this cult of the dead. Although in the process of mummification the internal organs were handled crudely, an opportunity was given of learning about the construction of the body. First the brain was extracted through the nostril; then the organs, except for the heart, were removed, the cavities emptied and filled with myrrh, cassia or other preservative; the openings were then sewn up, and the body, except for the head, soaked in sodium carbonate for seventy days. The head with the features intact was preserved by a thick resin. The corpse was then dried, dressed with resin, salt and fat, neatly swathed with linen and laid to rest in a coffin. The organs were carefully wrapped and placed in jars, or marked with the sign of their guardian god and returned to the body.

The Egyptians also gained some knowledge of anatomy from the custom of sacrificing animals, especially as signs and omens were looked for in the internal organs, the liver, the blood and even the urine. The Babylonians paid particular attention to the liver, which they thought was the source of the blood and the seat of the soul. Clay models have been found with special markings showing how they read the omens in accordance with the structure of the liver.

So in Babylonia and Egypt arose the first picture, blurred though it was, of how the bodies of men and animals were constructed.

Fact and Fantasy

Because of their general ignorance the Egyptians made many wild guesses about their medical problems. It was as though a modern man with no training in mechanics were asked to make a guess at the way in which a motor-car kept moving.

They could see that the body lived in a constant process of activity and change; but how exactly did it work? They knew that air was breathed in through the nose, and they decided that it must pass through the heart to leave the body through the anus; objects were often seen and heard simultaneously, so there must be a direct connection between the eye and the ear; the heart, the womb and the stomach gave rise to peculiar, unpredictable sensations, so they invested

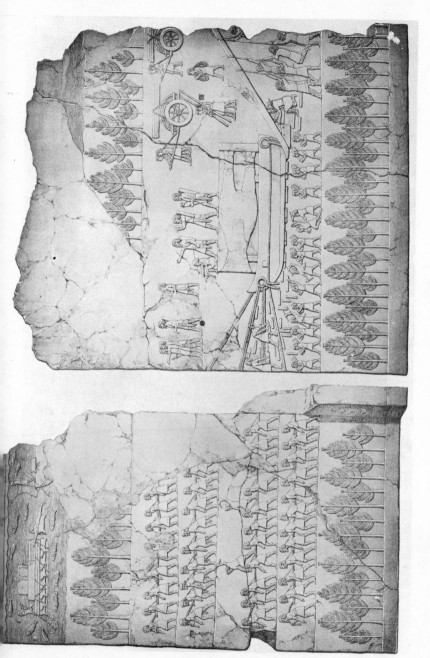

Assyrians moving a winged bull.

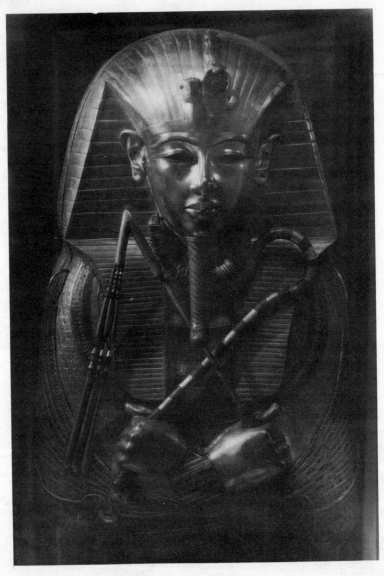

The gold coffin of Tut-Ankh-Amon.

them with moods and appetites which had to be satisfied for fear that they would wander restless and angry all over the body. When the heart stopped beating, life ended; so they reasoned that the heart was the centre of all thought and feeling. As the brain appeared to be connected through the skull with the nostrils and had no obvious function, it could only serve the purpose of expelling mucus from the nose. The organs such as the eyes, ears and stomach could survive only if they were fed by a constant supply of air and blood through the many vessels and tubes in the body. What happens when a person faints? The Egyptian physician explains to his students: "The heart does not speak—the vessels of the heart are dumb, there being no perception of them under thy fingers."

The Egyptians believed that every limb and organ was under the control of specific gods; each part of the body had its patron. An incantation from the famous Berlin Papyrus gives a list: "Thy arm is Horus, the other is Seth, thy navel is the Morning Star, thy leg is Isis . . ."

As in primitive times, the main theory of the origin of disease was that an evil demon had possessed the unfortunate body; and the aim of treatment was therefore to win over the gods to keep the demon away or to expel him by using the traditional spells, incantations and charms.

The priests practised innumerable rites for keeping the people in good health and curing them of sickness. They dominated the administration of medical relief, because illness was believed to be a form of punishment for sins; an Egyptian afflicted with blindness begins his prayer for mercy by declaring: "I am a man who swore falsely by Ptah, Lord of Truth; and he caused me to behold darkness by day."

Potions and Prayers

The ancient papyri are full of descriptions of such prayers and magic formulas; some are directed against the evils of drunkenness and diseases of childhood. Child-birth received special attention; hymns were sung over the bricks on which women knelt when in labour, and statuettes of goddesses and women helpers were in attendance. The special goddess of maternity was supposed to have given birth to the world; she was modelled with the features of a pregnant hippopotamus standing on her hind legs; in one paw she held the hieroglyph that meant "protection", and in the other, the sign of life.

The priest-physicians who recited the prayers and spells usually gave physical treatment as well, sometimes by the simple placing of hands on the patient; but there were also much more complicated practices.

Drugs and ointments were frequently used, and these also had to be applied with the necessary recitation by the doctor. As much of the medical literature of Egypt is given to recording such spells as to describing the diseases they were treating. While the priest-physician was interceding for the patient, he would speak for him in these typical words: "Come, Remedy. Come thou who expellest evil things in my stomach and in these my limbs! The spell is powerful over the ailment. Repeat it backwards!" Or, as the magical numbers were four and seven, it was repeated four or seven times. Very often the spell was more powerful than the ailment because of the psychological effect that it produced in the mind of the patient through the elaborate ritual of words, intonation of voice and gestures.

The practical remedies prescribed in the medical papyrus show a wide knowledge of drugs and herbs. There were recipes for all conditions: for constipation and for diarrhoea, for fastening loose teeth and for improving sight. And the drugs were given in different forms: in pills, enemas, suppositories, fumigations and inhalations. Just as the modern bottle of medicine has its additional touch of colour or flavour, so the ancient drugs had their appropriate spell.

Some of the ingredients of a prescription were brought together simply for their supposed magical value, such as the prescription for baldness, which contained the backbone of a raven, burnt hoof of an ass and the fat of a black snake. Many drugs derived from animals were bizarre and disgusting, often including blood and dung; the object was to make the potions so distasteful to the indwelling demons that they would prefer to come out rather than stay in the body. But there were many drugs such as minerals, vegetable extracts, gentian, castor oil and opium, which contained astringent and medicinal qualities so useful that they are still prescribed today.

It is amusing to note the recommendations often placed at the end of prescriptions: "this was very good", "excellent", "always success-ful", reminiscent of the puffs for patent medicines which appear in newspapers and magazines bearing unsolicited testimonials from Mrs X, Mr Y, and Dr X!

Their use of varied and elaborate remedies can be partly accounted for by the large number of Egyptian specialists. Each part of the body was under the care of specialists, such as eye-specialists, ear-specialists, heart specialists, internal organ specialists, and those with the picturesque title of Guardian Shepherd of the Anus. These specialists had their particular spells and incantations, but the people also put their faith in the support of charms against illness. The rich had their beads of gold and precious stones, and the poor had to rely on less impressive amulets made of linen sometimes containing the magic formulas. As with the spells, their use was governed by a complicated set of rules.

Such were the methods of treatment employed by the Egyptian priest-physicians. The papyri dealt with common diseases such as appendicitis, arthritis and gout. Even the most obviously natural phenomena, like disease of the eye or a snake-bite, were treated with the same distortion of reality by the overlying concept of magic.

The School of Practice

The Egyptians soon learnt from experience, however, that a broken bone could not be mended merely by a magic word written on an amulet, and magico-religious medicine was therefore devoted mainly to forms of sickness and disorder that did not require surgical inter-vention.

Surgical help was certainly needed in accidents and injuries. The building of cities and a new civilisation protected man from the dangers of attack by wild animals, but increased the risk of accidents from other causes. Injuries through accidents were frequent in Ancient Egypt, and they were often connected with the type of work the victim did.

The skulls of Egyptian women commonly show traces of serious ulceration, which was undoubtedly caused by their having to carry heavy water-jars; and however painful it was, they could not escape this duty.

We know from the works of Egyptian sculptors and other artists that the overseers of workers and slaves carried whips, not merely for ornament. The medical treatises, however, make no reference to the treatment of flesh wounds or others caused by the whip; no doubt the injury suffered was considered part of the punishment.

Again, although they are not mentioned, there must have been serious accidents in mining the precious copper and gold with which Egypt advanced her might. The human beings who were used as miners, however, could not have been valued less. Diodorus, a Greek historian of the time of the Ptolemies, described how the Kings of Egypt sent condemned prisoners and prisoners of war, together with their families, to work in the mines "naked and fettered", old and young alike, where they slaved until they dropped dead from exhaustion; they looked upon death as more desirable than life.

The fighting man, however, was not so easily replaced, and it is significant that the most rational treatise discovered, the Edwin Smith Papyrus, deals with a large variety of wounds including fractures, broken skulls, dislocations, smashed heads and similar injuries doubtless sustained in battle.

The Egyptians and Babylonians have confirmed in their tablets and plaques commemorating their victories what the Bible tells us of neighbouring races constantly warring with each other; the Hittites, the Assyrians, the Israelites and the Egyptians seemed always to be smiting one another, and the thrusting of bronze spears and swords could do much damage; so surgeons had a large amount of material for checking theory and practice. Embalmed bodies show many examples of fractured bones, almost always in the forearm near the wrist—which suggests the arm being raised in battle to ward off a blow to the head.

There was clearly no time on the field of battle for long-winded spells, and the Edwin Smith Papyrus shows that surgeons treated wounded persons with skill. The Papyrus described the treatment of forty-eight types of wounds of the head, neck, thorax, spine and limbs. The systematic arrangement of the book shows that it was intended to be a text-book of surgery. The document is incomplete, since it begins with injuries of the head and ends with an unfinished account of a sprain of the spinal column, omitting wounds of the abdomen and lower limbs.

It is clear that the surgeon first studied the injury carefully and decided on the most appropriate treatment before he started to operate. The qualities that made bronze suitable for tools and weapons also made it useful for medical instruments, and the surgeon had at his disposal a wide selection of knives, probes, forceps and surgical saws: better equipped than his predecessors, he was encouraged to make great advances in his practice.

The art of forecasting the course of the disease is also developed in the Edwin Smith Papyrus. In most cases the favourable prognosis was expressed in the words: "I will cure the disease." If the prognosis was doubtful, the formula was, "Nothing can be done in this case", and if unfavourable, "The patient will die". This was far removed from relying on the whims and passions of unpredictable gods and demons, and showed a keen sense of observation and a cool analysis of the patient's condition.

Just as there had to be a rational approach to building cities and dams and controlling floods, so in medicine the physicians made serious efforts to grasp the reality behind the phenomena of ill health. They were handicapped by the misconceptions they held, such as the sacred character of the liver, but their approach to the patient was in general practical and realistic.

They observed the sick person carefully, noting the slightest change in colour, expression and physical responses during the course of an illness. They studied the various parts of the body, the faeces, urine and discharges; they watched the temperature and felt the pulse. They also asked patients to move certain parts of the body to see if they had control over the muscles, and so were helped to diagnose conditions such as injury of the spinal column.

They classified over two hundred and sixty diseases; the causes of most of these, however, were unknown, and the symptom was usually identified with the disease. The "text-books", which introduced some order for the first time, were handed down from generation to generation, slavishly following a recognised form. For example, a gynaecological case would be entered firstly with the title: "Remedy for a woman who suffers from . . ."; then a list of her symptoms and the diagnosis: "Thou shalt say concerning it . . . the uterus has gone up (or down, is biting or restless)"; then the treatment: "Thou shalt do against it . . ."

Sometimes the doctor who had originally written the treatise would conclude the statement with a prognosis, "With this ailment I will contend", or, "This I will cure"; or, infrequently—but when said it amounted to a sentence of death—"Against this I can do nothing." A fatalistic attitude, in striking contrast to the modern contention that while there is life there is hope.

At some periods in Egyptian medical practice, there was clearly a distinction between the priest and the physician, as a poignant little poem indirectly testifies:

> Seven days from yesterday I have not seen my beloved,
> And sickness hath crept over me,
> And I am become heavy in my limbs,
> And am unmindful of mine own body.
> If the master-physicians come to me,
> My heart hath no comfort of their remedies.
> And the magicians, no resource is in them;
> My malady is not diagnosed. . . .
> Better for me is my beloved than any remedies.

From the anonymous generations of healers, Egyptian tradition has named one clearly defined personality, Imhotep, "One who brings peace". He was famed during his life for his abilities as a doctor and as an architect, poet and a wise counsellor to his king. Imhotep became immortalised as the God of Healing, and to the Egyptians he was the personification of the best in what has always been considered the noblest of professions.

Exchange of Knowledge

The river Nile was not only the source of plenty for the Egyptians, but it was also the great highway along which came the stream of commerce and culture from other parts of the world. From Egypt went the papyrus and handicrafts, and also her wisdom to colour and enrich much of the philosophical and scientific thought of the outside world; into Egypt came a selection of goods from Crete,

Babylonia, Assyria, India and from as far east as China. The peoples who came with their treasure along the well-travelled caravan routes and waterways brought with them the customs of their own civilisations; in Egypt there was a concentration of the experience of mankind.

Some of these cross-currents had a stronger influence than others; from the knowledge we have it is evident that the ancient Hindu civilisation was probably the most advanced in surgery, carrying out every known method of that time, including plastic surgery. They also introduced novel ways of training medical students by experimenting on animals, which is the groundwork of scientific teaching. Students studied and also practised on plants and hollow stalks of water-lilies or large veins of leaves, learning how to use their instruments deftly in puncturing and lancing. The next stage was experiment on the bodies and veins of animals. They also practised in opening gourds, cucumbers and leather bags filled with water, to get the feel of incising organs of the human body which contained fluid. Dead animals and flexible models were used for practise for the major operations.

From Babylonia the Egyptians learnt about medical consultations and how to relate symptoms to particular complaints. As Herodotus wrote: "They bring out their sick to the market place . . . then those who pass by the sick person confer with him about the disease, to discover whether they have themselves been afflicted with the same disease as the sick person, or seen others so afflicted; thus the passers-by confer with him, and advise him to have recourse to the same treatment as that by which they have escaped a similar disease, or as they have known to cure others."

Babylonia also set the example for a code of medical ethics, including a sliding scale of fees which the physician could charge. For a patrician the charge for treating a wound or opening an abscess of the eye with a bronze lancet was ten shekels of silver; for a poor man or a servant it was two to five shekels. But just as the rewards were more attractive for treating the wealthy, so the punishments for bad results were more severe: when the doctor caused the loss of a patient's life or eye, he had his hands cut off if the victim were a patrician, and he had to pay compensation if the man were a slave.

China introduced the concept of state medical examinations, and the physician's salary was fixed according to the standard he had reached at the end of the year.

At this period, civilisation was most advanced in countries with hot climates; and Egypt benefited from the experience of other peoples with similar medical problems. Swamp and marsh had to be properly drained, the refuse of large towns disposed of, and serious attention paid to the prevalence of flies and rats and the dangers of infection; adequate supplies of pure water had to be provided.

Their knowledge of mathematics, geometry and engineering construction helped the Egyptians to find satisfactory solutions to some of these problems, and so reduce the spread of epidemics such as malaria, cholera, plague and unpleasant worm and eye infections which even today harass the dwellers of the Nile valley; the medical problems were typical of an area subject to yearly inundations along a river-course.

From the Cretan civilisation, the Egyptians learnt the use of copper pipes for sanitation and for collecting rain-water. Excavations of the temples show arrangements for baths and lavatories. The great cities of the Euphrates and the Tigris were probably more advanced in their sanitation. India at this period was also well provided with means for a pure water supply and the disposal of refuse. Indian physicians practised inoculation against smallpox, and used antidotes and inoculation against snake bites; they realised there was a connection between outbreaks of bubonic plague and the presence of rats.

Some of the outstanding achievements of Egyptian social hygiene have reached us through the Mosaic Laws, the code of a small nation, the Jews, who lived in partial slavery to the Egyptians during their wanderings from their original homeland along the edge of the Arabian desert. The Jews worshipped only one God: a God who they maintained was the source of life and of sickness and death.

The Jews played an important part in helping to free Egyptian medical thought from its obsession with devils and "evil eyes". In the Jewish Talmud the rules of social hygiene and the treatment of sickness are interlocked with religious concepts. The Jews taught, to the lasting benefit of mankind, that cleanliness and Godliness were one. A further advance on orthodox Egyptian thought was the Jewish

insistence on the rights and responsibilities of all members of the
community to observe the laws of hygiene; to this small race, which
had suffered so heavily under the Pharaohs, we are indebted for one
of the most humane and healthful injunctions: "Six days shalt thou
labour and on the seventh shalt thou rest." For partly religious and
partly social incentives, the people were recommended not to drink
an excess of beer, nor over-indulge in sex nor to practise perversions,
and they were instructed how to eat clean food and guard against
contagious diseases.

The Egyptians adopted many of these excellent precepts. The citizen washed and anointed himself daily; he protected his food and
drink from contamination by flies and other sources of infection; he
slept under mosquito nets and washed his clothes regularly.

He went to some extreme to keep himself clean internally as well
as outwardly; there may have been a religious origin in the custom
of evacuating the intestinal tract with emetics and enemas on three
consecutive days in the month, or perhaps it was believed that diseases
were caused by excess of food.

Greek observers formed a high opinion of the standard of health
of the Egyptians, which was certainly due to their rational rules of
living. Diodorus wrote of them: "The whole manner of life was so
evenly ordered that it would appear as though it had been arranged
according to the rules of health by a learned physician." Herodotus
said that the Egyptians were the healthiest of all men, next to the
Libyans.

Egypt's Contribution to Medicine

Man's reasoning powers, constantly brought into action with the
everyday struggle of existence, had made some headway against the
restraining influence of age-old superstitions. It was true that many
sensible practices carried out by the individual and the community
were bound up with solemn ritual associated with the gods in their
gold and marble temples, and it would be difficult to unravel the
thread of common sense from the intricate patterns of superstition
with which it was interwoven.

It can be said that Egyptian medicine advanced greatly in the
rational treatment of surgical wounds and in personal and social

hygiene, but the Egyptians were hampered by their lack of knowledge of the body, and by the artificial division that had arisen between worker by hand and worker by brain. Theoretical ideas were evolved in the semi-darkness of the temples, far from everyday practice which could have led physicians further into the field of real experience and new discoveries. Scarcely any attention was paid to the health and well-being of slaves in comparison with the importance attached by medicine and religion to the glory of the rulers in life and death.

For a thousand years after Egypt had achieved the best of her scientific and social development, this conservative dogma continued. Science and medicine could make no great step forward when new ways of living, new experiments and new thinking were discouraged. Towards the end of the Egyptian empire of the last period it was as though their obsessive fear would become a reality, and the darkness of the tomb would spread and engulf the land of the living.

Nevertheless, Ancient Egypt has bequeathed more than the huge monuments designed to last for eternity. Her wisdom, her brave attempts at rational thought in the midst of a world of mysterious phenomena, her rules of social hygiene and the logic of her science —all these have lived on through the newer civilisations which arose. And if today we are still bewitched, as were the Egyptians, by too much faith in a bottle of medicine or in the casting of a horoscope, we honour them for starting man on the long road of rational thought and action.

Chapter Three

GREEK MEDICINE

A New Age Begins

THE Egyptian Empire was doomed: condemned by its dependence on tradition and its failure to introduce new methods in agriculture and industry.

The tribute extracted from conquered countries was wasted in useless luxuries and the elaborate religious customs dedicated mainly to the cult of the dead. The Egyptians had gained advantage over other peoples because of their superior knowledge and their use of weapons and tools of bronze. These weapons were put into the hands of great numbers of mercenaries, who in time turned them against their Egyptian taskmasters.

The great empires of the Bronze Age suffered an eclipse about 1200 B.C. Egypt, Babylon, Persia, China—all sank into a dark and uninspired way of life; the arts and sciences repeated the old traditional pattern. Some momentous change in man's way of living was necessary to release the potential streams of energy held back by this narrow existence.

The key that opened up the gates to the new era of expansion was forged of iron. Lying so abundantly in the earth, it proved to be a far more potent servant to man's needs than bronze. Plentiful supplies of tools gave added power to the slave hands, who could now be engaged on a far greater scale than before on the necessary work of clearing trees, breaking up the earth for more intensive farming and digging channels for drainage. Eager hands seized the tools and set to work to produce an abundance of food and grain essential for the expansion of society.

The use of iron spread from about 1200 B.C., but it had come too late to save the declining Empires of India, China and especially Egypt.

The potentialities of this new commodity could best be exploited by a people who were only just breaking free from barbarism, and were therefore not bound by the conventions of a rigid Bronze Age civilisation; it was also necessary to have a good coastline so that the flow of goods could be easily and cheaply transported along the trade lines to other lands.

Of the peoples in the Near East and Mediterranean lands, the Greeks alone had both these advantages, and so they were able to leap forward and for a time lead the world in the development of all creative work, art, philosophy, medicine and the sciences.

There was no fundamental change in the slave system, but with the introduction of iron, the new Greek Empire was able to expand the economy, so that for a time the underlying difficulties were eased.

The Greeks, keeping ahead of other nations, had to exercise great ingenuity, and they responded magnificently to the challenge of their time by advancing the sciences of mathematics, physics, chemistry and astronomy, and creating the glory of Greek philosophy and art. Cities and ports grew rapidly, and teemed with people of all classes, creating new problems of living together in health and good citizenship; medical theory and practice, evolving in this time of profound change and activity, progressed rapidly with the other sciences.

The School of Rational Medicine

Greek medicine produced three main schools which made varying contributions to medical practice.

The philosophical school of medicine studied sickness and disease on the basis of theory isolated from practice.

A second school of medical treatment was the successor to the ancient mystico-magical practices, and was conducted in the Greek temples of Aesculapius, the God of Healing.

The rational school of medicine, based on the teaching of Hippocrates, was influenced by the methods used in dealing with the new problems created in the growing cities, the centres of commerce and in the extensive military adventures of the empire. Hippocratic thought profoundly affected medical ideas for over 1,000 years, from the sixth century B.C. to the fourth century A.D.

The wise Greeks had already learnt that if navigators were to reach new lands, and farmers to wrest more riches from the soil, prayers were not enough: they studied the stars and extended their knowledge of mathematics and geography to further these practical aims, and the results reinforced their scepticism about magic omens and divine revelations. Some doctors arrived at similar conclusions. They sat at the bedside and carefully observed the patient. As the new botanists and zoologists studied plants, animals and minerals, classifying them according to their types and forms, and not, as had been customary, on the basis of mystical names and symbols, so doctors studied man, introducing some system in their medical inspection, which led to more rational methods of treatment.

Hippocrates, honoured in all the history books as "Father of Clinical Medicine", is something of a legendary figure, but the works of his followers over a period of five or six centuries are well known, and the famous collection of their medical writings is based on the manuscripts in the library of Alexandria, where they were carefully copied and kept for posterity. The scientific brilliance of Greek rational medicine was for a time obscured by the darkness of the Middle Ages in Europe, but, as with all of man's decisive victories over ignorance, it has outlasted the doctrines which served only to stifle progress.

The great strength of the Hippocratic school was the deep affection for humanity and respect for the art of healing, expressed so well in their famous maxim: "Where there is love of man, there is also love for the art." To the conscientious doctor, they were two sides of the same coin: they could not be separated. This concern for the patient permeated their medical practice. All the unnatural phenomena of mysticism, magic and astrology were put on one side as impediments to rational scientific thinking about the problem of the illness.

Recognising the Illness

The bedside manner of the Hippocratic doctor was no mere formality; he kept a close watch on the developing course of the illness. He paid attention to the way the patient lay in bed, how he breathed and slept, his pulse and his temperature. He made a thoughtful analysis of his pains and the movements of his body. On the basis of observation and reasoning, it became possible to narrow down the causes of diseases and classify them according to diagnosis, prognosis. and response to treatment.

Many of the Greek clinical records and descriptions of cases have remained classics for our own day. They described diseases such as tuberculosis, child-bed fever, epilepsy, mumps and malaria with a perspicacity and simple directness which cannot be improved.

Tuberculosis was not a new disease even in Ancient Greece; the watchful doctors described accurately the shivering fever, the profuse sweating and severe chilling of the extremities, the wasting, the loss of appetite and the characteristic cough and sputum. Such sufferers, they wrote, have "bright eyes, a smooth skin of whitish or of reddish hue, and wing-like shoulder-blades".

One among many graphic case-histories is that of Thasus, the wife of Philinus, who died of child-bed fever on the twentieth day after the birth of her child. The familiar symptoms are registered; the shivering attacks, delirium and convulsions leading to the fatal end.

There is an impressive honesty about the manner in which the medical failures as well as the successes are recorded, with the detachment of genuine scientific study. The doctors are aware of their limitations, and for the sake of the art of medicine, they record their cases exactly; out of the forty-two cases reported in the writings, twenty-five had fatal results. "But," said the author of one of the case histories, "I have written this down deliberately believing it is invaluable to learn of unsuccessful experiments and to know the causes of their failure." This approach did not exclude a human sympathy towards the patient, who was handled with care and thoughtfulness.

The accurate description and classification of these clinical cases testifies to the powerful reasoning of the Hippocratic doctors.

The Sick Man in His Setting

Just as there are today, there were then conflicting theories about disease, all with their fervent supporters. The Hippocratic school was particularly critical of the neighbouring school of Cnidos, which adhered to an old tradition of treating only the organ which appeared to be the one mainly affected—an approach encouraging an elaborate therapy with little or no regard to the fundamental causes of disease.

The rational school of medicine had moved so far from the demon-ridden days of the witch-doctor, that doctors were able to step back and look at the sick man as he really was, a human being in his particular setting; they realised the importance of that setting, and they were prepared to consider which of its components may have contributed to his ill health.

When Silenus, a young man who "lived on The Broadway", was suddenly taken ill with fever, his illness was ascribed to "the consequences of exertion, drinking, and unseasonable exercises". Again, in one of the Hippocratic text-books called *Airs, Waters and Places*, the physician is advised to study the background of his patients; he must note the climate, the situation, the water supply and the type of vegetation where his patients live. The author had travelled abroad, and in the second half of the book he makes the point that races differ in their habits and well-being according to the variation in climate.

An example of the author's scepticism about divine speculation is shown in his account of upper-class Scythians, many of whom were afflicted with impotence. Although he attributes this to excessive horse-riding, he is clear on one point; the condition was not divine in origin, for, "if this were true, it would not attack the most highborn and wealthy Scythians alone, but all alike; in fact, rather those with small possessions who do not offer sacrifices to the gods"; and he concludes with a Parthian shot—"if indeed the gods take pleasure in the homage of men and grant them favours in return".

There is a present day adage: "Tell me what you eat and I'll tell you what you are." The Greeks did not go as far as this, but they did pay particular attention to the effect of diet and the water-supply on the human body, and with their customary wisdom they made an acute observation which can well serve as a guide today: "Old persons endure fasting more easily; next, adults; young persons not nearly so well; and most especially infants, and of them, such as are of a particularly lively spirit."

Almost the seven ages of man, in one of the most pithy and precise of Greek aphorisms.

Forecasting the Course of Illness

Broad as was this approach to clinical medicine, the Hippocratic school employed yet another method which added to the value of their treatment. They reasoned that man's disorders are not an unchanging condition: men fall ill through some cause, and progress towards recovery or death. It is not enough to recognise and name the process; the doctor must watch its development and apply his art and skill to influence the trend of events.

By this careful training in observation, they attempted to forecast the likely course of the disease, having considered its history and present state. The reputation of the Hippocratic doctors was particularly enhanced by their skill in prognosis.

In particular, they learnt a great deal from their study of acute fevers, which were widespread in a country with a hot climate and with only an elementary knowledge of communal hygiene. Fevers, more than any other ailment, follow a recognisable course, and the Greek doctors soon grasped the theory of crisis which they described as developing through three stages: beginning, height and decline, with sometimes death as the outcome.

A good doctor observes the object of his study with the keen eye of an artist, and it was certainly an artist's pen that described the famous Hippocratic sign of approaching death:

"The nose sharp, eyes hollow, temples sunken, ears cold and contracted and lobes everted; the skin about the face hard, tense and wizened, and the colour of the whole face yellow or dark; these symptoms being particularly dangerous when they were associated with the hands searching through empty air, picking nap from the bedclothes, plucking at particles and snatching chaff from the walls."

Nearer to our own times, the supreme artist Shakespeare gave to the Hostess in *Henry V* almost these very words to describe Falstaff's end: "I saw him fumble with the sheets, and play with flowers, and smile upon his fingers' end, I knew there was but one way; for his nose was as sharp as a pen, and 'a babbled of green fields."

The combined experience of generations of doctors trained in the Hippocratic tradition was crystallised in aphorisms like these, which have not lost their truth with the passing centuries:

"When sleep puts an end to delirium it is a good sign."

"In every disease it is a good sign when the patient's intellect is sound and he enjoys his food; the opposite is a bad sign."

"Old men generally have less illness than young men, but such complaints that become chronic in old men generally last until death."

"Those who are attacked by tetanus either die in four days, or if they survive this period, they recover."

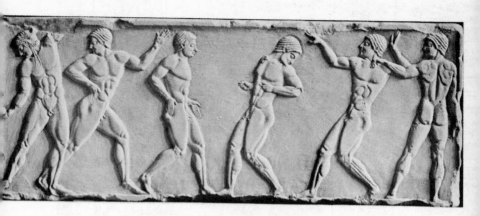

Athletes of the Ancient World.

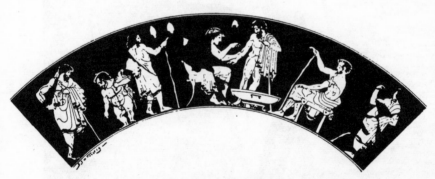

A Greek clinic.

Temple of Aesculapius.

"If diarrhoea attacks a consumptive patient it is a fatal symptom."
The doctors who made these comments in forecasting the course
of a disease had no misconceptions about indwelling demons and
occult influences; they saw that here was a life and death struggle in
the body between its innate tendency to right itself, and the harmful
agent which was upsetting the body's natural balance.

Treating Illness

It was the Greeks who gave humanity the profoundly simple and
sensible belief in the healing power of nature. The doctor therefore
adopted the expectant line of treatment, assisting the patient's natural
resistance by simple remedies such as a course of good food, fresh
air, massage and hydrotherapy, and purgation to keep his system
wholesome. The famous Greek cult of "the body beautiful" was based
on the recognised health value of gymnastics, exercises and bathing.

The Greeks taught the excellence of moderation in all things, and
the recommended diet for patients did not go further than a few
simple prescriptions such as barley gruel, which was named often,
and a general liquid diet in cases of fever and wounds. As in very
ancient times, honey was thought to have healing qualities, but drugs
were used cautiously. This compares significantly with the medical
treatment of previous ages when magic rites and sacrifices were inex-
tricably mixed with great varieties of drugs, herbs and potions ranging from the pleasant to the disgusting.

This restraint in prescribing drugs was based on the general approach of the Hippocratic doctors, and not on any lack of knowledge; a great variety of plants were being discovered in the course
of a progressive agricultural and botanical science. Discorides, a Greek
army surgeon who, like many of his colleagues, travelled and studied
in the course of his medical work, compiled a text-book classifying
over 600 plants; his book was in popular use for over 2,000 years—
a record for any medical work. Almost 100 of these plant prescriptions are in use today. This harvest of information was not the fruit
of one man's labour; Greece at that flourishing time had many minor
Discorides: midwives, chemists, veterinary surgeons, root-gatherers
and others who in the course of their work collected herbs and plants.

After all is said, the Hippocratic Collection of Writings themselves speak best of the quality of the rational treatment of their times:

"Do not disturb a patient either during or just after a crisis, and try no experiments, neither with purges nor with other irritants; leave him alone."

"For extreme diseases extreme strictness of treatment is most efficacious."

"It is better to give no treatment in cases of hidden cancer: treatment causes speedy death; to omit treatment is to prolong life."

The Collections open with a brief statement which underlines the dignity, wisdom and humility of these ancient Greek physicians:

"Life is short, the Art long, occasion sudden, experience fallible, and judgment difficult. Not only must the physician show himself prepared to do what is needed; but he must make the patient, the attendants, and the surrounding circumstances co-operate with him."

Good Practice and Bad Theory

The achievements of the Hippocratic school had in some ways been negative rather than positive. They had cleared the air as never before of the fog of superstition and fear surrounding disease. With logic that would not be out of date in the twentieth century, they challenged the witch-mutterings on the most dread of all diseases, epilepsy. "This disease is no more divine than any other. It has a natural cause just as other diseases have. Men think it is divine merely because they do not understand it. But if they called everything divine which they did not understand, why, there would be no end of divine things." But it was not enough to criticise ancient misconceptions; the void left by the destruction of superstitious beliefs had to be filled with new ideas, otherwise new errors would creep in. In fact, the Greek physicians, like other scientists, were subject to various influences. They were moving forward under the impact of the exciting new times they lived in; they had inherited much knowledge of mathematics, astronomy and medical practice from the old civilisations of Egypt and Judea; but they were restricted by their ignorance of anatomy, physiology and pathology, and by the absence of a coherent and rational philosophy.

They drew a picture of the internal workings of the body which was at times as far from reality as the imagined world of a blind man.

They thought, for instance, that arteries were full of air, since they were found to be empty at death; they imagined that arteries came from the heart, and veins from the liver; and for 2,000 years this error was perpetuated. They could not differentiate clearly between nerves, tendons, and blood vessels. The process of child-birth seemed in particular to be veiled to the Greeks, and their treatment of sterility was inspired by mysticism rather than rational thought. They considered that the womb had two pouches and concluded that the one on the right was reserved for male children and the one on the left for females.

Hippocratic medicine scored no great success in the realm of theory; but in practising the art of surgery made some spectacular steps forward. One of its most revealing axioms was that "War is the only proper school for the surgeon".

Certainly these Greek surgeons learnt in practice about the bones and joints, from all the mishaps that could befall men in war or sport. Also they obtained useful anatomical demonstrations at the great sports arenas, where nude youths took part in every type of physical exercise.

They were able to distinguish between simple and compound fractures, and could gauge the approximate time it would take the bone to rejoin. They could show accurately where and how the injured limb should be placed and were helped in their work by improved types of instruments, special apparatus and the excellent co-operation of medical teams. The Collection describes the procedure for reducing a dislocation of the hip joint, a procedure typical of their technical standards. The patient is suspended from a cross-beam, and when all the necessary preparations are made, "A well-trained man of considerable strength" clasps his forearm around the patient's groin, and then both are suspended so that the weights of patient and assistant can help to force the head of the thigh-bone back into position. The surgeons must truly have earned the confidence of the patients to be able to gain their co-operation in these difficult and very painful manœuvres.

A special treatise written on "Fractures, dislocations, and wounds of the head" reveals a knowledge of surgical technique which compares favourably with modern methods. For example, they recommended trephining in injuries of the head to relieve pressure on the brain; they concluded that resting an injured limb was more helpful than bandaging, and their surgical practice progressed to such a state of refinement that for certain cases of fracture of the jaw the use of gold wire was recommended, although it is indeed unlikely that this was ever used for treating fractures suffered by slaves or poor citizens.

The Greeks knew nothing of germs, yet they learnt from experience to use pure or boiled water in treating wounds; and their instructions to surgeons might have come direct from a modern text-book: "Have the nails neither to exceed nor come short of the finger tips . . . all operations to be practised with each hand and with both together."

From the spirit of integrity which shines through all they wrote, one thing is crystal clear: the doctors of the Hippocratic school practised what they preached.

Big Cities Create Big Problems

The Greeks were busily founding a modern empire on the soil of the past. With the growing cities at home and the new dependencies abroad, new public health problems arose: the incessant demands for improved sanitation, good water-supply, drainage and sewage disposal, and proper burial facilities—demands that had to be met so that industry and commerce, even life itself, could advance unhindered.

When people think of classical Greece, they remember its glory, and picture the cities such as Athens with its magnificent public buildings, and its wide squares graced by fountains, just as foreigners often visualise London as St Paul's and the Houses of Parliament. But Ancient Athens, as important in its time as London is today, has to be seen as a whole, especially when the health and well-being of its inhabitants are considered.

Most of its people lived in dark and mean houses in narrow, twisting streets. The ordinary housewife had to go to the street fountain for water. Water was a problem for Greek sanitary engineers because the soil was dry. Underground aqueducts were constructed to bring water down from the mountains, and the large wells that were sunk had to go very deep. The housewife had to cope with primitive sanitary arrangements; the latrine in the house was of a simple type and she had to flush it with slop water which was drained into sewers under the street.

The character of the problems raised in these closely packed cities was a challenge and a stimulus to the practical school of Greek medicine. The germs of infectious diseases were the main trouble-makers, yet their existence was unknown. The doctors did not know the cause of cholera, dysentery or typhoid, or how these diseases spread with such fearful rapidity; and they attributed these alarming occurrences to sudden changes in the atmosphere, the disturbances created by war, or to the wrath of gods and demons. Often enough the people threw aside all reason and fell back on magic and religious rites to combat a terrifying epidemic, as they did at Numa, in the eighth century B.C., when a man dressed in a goatskin was driven from the city: the original scapegoat, perhaps. When the epidemic subsided, the preventive measures took the form of repeating the practice twice yearly. Three hundred years later it is recorded that an epidemic affecting women was ended by burying alive a vestal virgin who had sinned. Ignorance and fear together have always impaired people's relations with one another, and it is disappointing to learn that in an age where there was so much logical thinking, people could be accused of deliberately spreading an epidemic with malice aforethought.

A little more rational, even if not based on any sound knowledge of plague, were the attempts to combat this disease, in the year 430 A.D., by building great fires in the streets of Athens. It was thought that in this way the polluted air could be purified, and so prevent contagion, which is the Greek word for "propagation".

Rational medicine, however, adopting the practical approach characteristic of the best achievements of Greek science, was making some headway in combating epidemics.

These doctors realised that the maintenance of good health was linked with clean water and sanitation, the destruction of tainted food, and the disposal of sewage and the burial of the dead outside the city limits. As in the practice of their clinical medicine, with the accent on observation, they came remarkably close to correct answers. They knew that rain water contained impurities and unless it was boiled, could produce bad odours, sore throats, coughs and hoarseness. They surmised that dust and flies played some part in spreading epidemics. And although they had no knowledge of the malarial parasite and the way it was introduced through the bite of mosquitoes, they knew malaria was in some way associated with marsh lands, and they made efforts to drain these unhealthy areas. Despite these preventive steps, the mosquito proved itself capable of undermining the constitution of this people who had surmounted so many other obstacles. Even today in a period of far greater medical knowledge, malaria still impoverishes the colonial peoples of an empire vaster than the Greeks ever dreamed of.

Greek Hygiene

Today, we frequently judge preventive health standards by the chances of survival offered to that most vulnerable being, the new-born infant. It is doubtful if this thought occurred to the Greeks, whose knowledge of infant care was meagre: on the contrary, infanticide of the weak or deformed was an accepted custom. The high death rate of infants, however, was mainly due to ignorance and the unhealthy conditions of living of the majority of the people. In dealing with another subject, Aristotle tells us, "Most babies die before the week is out; consequently they are not named until that time because there is then more hope for survival".

For those that did survive, there was the very considerable attraction of developing a physically fit body by training in the public gymnasia and baths, and by taking part in the games and sports; they aimed at achieving the positive good health which the Greeks equated with beauty. Another side of this cult was that it undoubtedly helped in developing that essential person, the soldier, and to further this, the Greek State emphasised the theme (to be taken up with greater emphasis by the Roman conquerors) of how glorious it is to die for one's country. The military campaigns indirectly promoted good health; army doctors, besides widening their surgical experience, considerably strengthened their practical knowledge in solving problems of disposing of refuse and sewage, and of burying the dead.

Different ages reach the peak of achievement in varying activities. We in Great Britain are proud that just over 100 years ago we appointed the first public medical officer of health. But 2,000 years ago the Greeks had developed sufficient understanding and public spirit to appoint well-paid and highly honoured physicians to supervise the health of districts and cities and treat the poor who could not pay the usual private fees. The people attended public surgeries, which were supported by local taxation, and these were like a modern health centre: medicine was dispensed and operations carried out. There were other public medical appointments; medical officers were attached to public schools, gymnasia and arenas, and some acted as medical advisers to local magistrates.

Above all, the Hippocratic school encouraged the concept of social hygiene, and one of this school, Diocles, wrote the first text-book on this subject, emphasising the need for good housing and sanitation, clean water, and clothing appropriate to the season; he stressed the rational approach to disease as opposed to priestcraft and belief in magic. He expounded the central theme of Greek medical thought —man was a being at one with nature, and the preservation of this harmony by healthy living and open-air cures for illness was natural and closest to the Greek conception of true hygiene.

The Greek World of Philosophy

The philosophers of Ancient Greece have come to share the immortality conferred by their own poets upon their gods and goddesses on Mount Olympus. They did indeed move and think in a world remote from the toiling slaves and subject peoples who were the main support of the Greek Empire.

The opening of the iron age stimulated an expansion in commerce and in the new realms of experiment and discovery. The intellectuals made considerable advances in the sciences of astronomy, mathematics and geometry, but this only tended to widen the gulf stretching between this small leisured class and the many who were engaged in manual labour. The philosophers declared that physical work and those who performed it were beneath their notice, and they in turn became more and more drawn into abstract theorising unchecked by practice. Plato, the leading philosopher, wrote: "The people are a third class, consisting of those who work with their own hands; they are not politicians and they have not much to live upon."

The steady supply of slave labour gave little encouragement for applying scientific thought to evolving new technical improvements or labour-saving devices; craftsmanship was regarded as the mark of servility, and the philosophers therefore withdrew, if not to Mount

Olympus, at least to a world of their own, where their heads often touched the clouds at the expense of their feet leaving *terra firma*.

For example, out of the practical observations that the school of mathematicians made on numbers and their fascinating possibilities, emerged a romantic belief in their magical properties. The Greeks did in fact learn to apply a systematic logic to conditions which they dealt with and mastered. But instead of paying tribute to the growth of man's reasoning powers in these achievements, they thought they had uncovered the qualities of ideal triangles and other mathematical figures existing outside of man's practical work, and the mathematicians concluded that they could find the answer to the riddle of the universe if only they manipulated the numbers correctly.

From such philosophical abstraction, any absurdity could be reasoned to be logical. The figure four appealed to the Greek thinkers as being especially potent. The four basic elements of fire, earth, air and water had four corresponding qualities—hot, dry, cold and moist. Also, the human body had its complement of four humours, blood, phlegm, yellow bile and black bile, which had similar qualities of heat, dryness and so on. The humours and qualities were associated with the different organs of the body, and they combined in different ways with varying effects on the person's health. A sick person, for example, might be suffering from too much of the qualities of hot and dry, indicating an overdose of yellow bile; too much of the cold and moist went with an increase in phlegm, often producing a phlegmatic temperament. Strangely enough, these early medical theories, based on misconceptions as they were, have nevertheless been echoed faintly in the modern view of endocrine and biochemical imbalances as the cause of illness.

Teacher and Pupil

The philosophers sat in their lofty halls and in an atmosphere of calm and dignity passed on the sum of their knowledge to a chosen fraternity. What happened to man in his physical life was considered unworthy of discussion; it was man's soul that was of importance, and that stayed in the bodily prison only for a time, and could pass from one to another. *The Republic*, Plato's greatest work, concerns itself with much ingenious argument about the way to manage men

—the caged souls in the perishable bodies; there was no thought for the management and control of the environment which made man's life what it was.

Plato had as a pupil, Aristotle, whose contribution to mankind was of practical value thousands of years after the Platonic theories had ceased to be of more than academic interest to universities and their students.

Aristotle had the true scientist's intense curiosity about all creatures, great and small. He pursued his inquiries about life along the seashores of Greece, studying and classifying the great varieties of fish, molluscs and plants, their construction and habits, with infinite care and patience. He assembled all the known facts about botany, zoology and physiology, and so gave medical science a firm basis on which to build further knowledge.

But Aristotle could not, in the philosophical field, free himself from the Platonic ideas, which his guide and teacher had impressed on him; namely, that some men were born to be slaves so that others, their masters, could live the intellectual life, studying philosophy, mathematics and theology. It was logical then to support and justify the system of slavery, for on this foundation free citizens (like Plato and Aristotle) could live in peaceful and fruitful contemplation. If everything in the state was so arranged in the best possible order, then the lesser organisation of parts and functions, the body, must likewise serve a perfect design. Much more thought was spent on divining the ideal purpose of each bodily organ than on studying seriously how it worked.

This attitude led even so profound a thinker as Aristotle to arrive at conclusions very far from reality. In his study of embryology, Aristotle noticed that the heart was the first part of the body to show a sign of life, and when it ceased to beat, life ended. He reasoned, therefore, that the heart must be the seat of intelligence; the brain acted merely to cool the heart. Aristotle accepted the philosophers' theory that the soul progressed from body to body, and he added his own interpretation that this soul (or psyche) was transmitted through the male; the female playing the passive and lesser role of providing the material habitation which, infused with life by the soul, created a new being.

Remote as all this philosophising was from the everyday life of the people, it was at times brought in to play a necessary part, just as did the religious teachings, in maintaining the *status quo*. From time to time the slave empires felt a shuddering in their foundations, as the people through desperation or hope tried to throw off their gigantic shackles. Then the philosophers were able to prove the value of their dialectic. Plato raised a mountain of logic to justify teaching the people, in times of stress, "a noble lie".

The Hold of Magic

While the most forward-looking of the Greeks were striving towards rational answers to their problems, particularly in the methods adopted by the practical school of medicine, a third force trailed behind in the mists of priestcraft and witchery, carrying on the ancient traditions of magical healing in the Greek temples dedicated to the God Aesculapius.

It was the function of the magico-mystical school of healing to connect the religious ideal of purification with bodily purification, and they tried to achieve this effect by strong suggestion coloured by the practice of magic rites.

The temples of healing stood in green groves beside springs of pure and medicinal waters. They were graceful and often magnificent, equipped with gymnasiums, stadiums, and theatres, and decorated with works of art by the finest masters. The stage was well set for medical treatment by suggestion.

The patient who came to the temple would receive a preliminary initiation by a specially trained priest-physician, who told of the previous successes of the God. The body and spirit were prepared by strict diet, omitting wines and certain types of food, by purgation, ritual bathing in the spring, and finally by prayers and the sacrifice of an animal, a cock or a ram. The patient, after final purification by a bath often accompanied by rhythmic massage, was ready finally for the climax of the treatment. During the night as he lay in the temple, he would be visited by the priest in the shape of the God himself, who administered advice to him if he was awake; if he was asleep, he was later convinced that the God had appeared in his dreams. The modern theories of Freud immediately come to mind

when one reads of dream interpretations and even the types of sug-
gestive treatment the priest prescribed, including catharsis, emetics
and blood-letting.

The grateful patient, frequently cured if his illness was of a psychological character, would give a thank-offering to the temple, in the
shape of a wax, silver or gold model of the afflicted part. Sometimes
a tablet giving the history of his case was suspended in the temple
as a lasting tribute to yet one more remarkable cure. In addition, he
would throw money into the healing waters of the spring.

The type of case and the mercenary methods of the priest are well
illustrated in the story of Hermo, of Pasos. It is written, "The God
cured him of his blindness, but when he refused to pay the honor-
arium to the sanctuary, the God made him blind again as a punishment. When he returned again and slept once more in the temple,
the God healed him again."

There is more than a hint of shrewd salesmanship under the priestly
manner in the story of the father of a dumb boy who had undergone
the usual initiation. When the father was asked, "Do you promise
to pay within a year the fees for the cure, if you obtain that for which
you have come?" he heard his son suddenly answer, "I do!" The
father asked the son to repeat the words, which he did, and so
was cured.

The Greek temple physicians had a large following, and undoubtedly there were genuine cures, including some cases of sterility
remedied by the active intervention of the priests. There were other
disorders, however, which would not yield to psycho-therapy, or to
its distortion into rites which were merely the old mumbo-jumbo
in Greek.

Aristophanes wrote, for the upper class of educated Greeks, his
comedy *Plutus* which satirised this temple treatment and enjoyed a
great popularity amongst the more sophisticated, who did not exert
themselves, however, to enlighten their more ignorant fellows.

Wisdom, Learning and Experience

These various schools of thought were not separate rivers meander-
ing in different lands; they were streams that met and mingled, and
they all flowed along the same bedrock of a slave society.

The philosophical schools of Plato and Aristotle reached some startling misconceptions about medicine, but it was at least of great value that they brought the subject into discussion among philosophers; the practical work of the doctor or scientist needed the inspiration of general discussion, just as theory becomes sterile when out of touch with practice.

The school of Hippocratic medicine took the first mature step towards practical treatment; they took a rational view of illness, and treated the patient objectively; but the abstract theories which they left standing at the front door crept in by the back when the need for some greater guide than immediate experience was required. Without theories of their own, they had to rely on the idealistic conceptions spun out of the intangible but ever-present magico-religious influences of the temple school.

The Doctors and the People

While the intellectuals disputed, people lived and toiled, sickened, suffered and died, from one generation to another, without any great change in the way they were treated medically.

Plato gives a vivid description of the medical profession in his time:

"There are physicians, and again there are physicians' assistants, whom we also speak of as physicians . . . all bear the name, whether freemen or slaves who gain their professional knowledge by watching their masters and obeying their directions in empiric fashion. . . . The slaves, to speak generally, are treated by slaves who pay them a hurried visit, or receive them in dispensaries. . . . A physician of this kind never gives a servant any account of his complaint, nor asks him for any; he gives some empiric injunction with an air of finished knowledge, in the brusque fashion of a dictator, and then is off in hot haste to the next ailing servant; that is how he lightens his master's medical labours for him."

Again, the Hippocratic school had some stringent criticism to make of certain types of doctors; they are compared with bad pilots whose ignorance is exposed only when they lose their ships in a violent gale: "When bad physicians, who comprise the vast majority, treat men who are suffering from no serious complaints (which are far more common than serious disease), their greatest blunders do not affect them seriously and so they are not shown up in their true colours to laymen; it is only when they meet with a severe, violent and dangerous illness, that their errors and want of skill become manifest to all."

The system which made such a vast difference between the life of one section of the community, as against the vast majority in the debased position of slaves and poor craftsmen, was bound to be reflected in a distorted form of medical treatment and an ill-balanced attitude to the patient.

However, the element of logic and clear thinking was at work in the best minds of Greece, and the Hippocratic oath which was enjoined on all true followers of this school embodied a humanity which outlived all that was unworthy in the State.

The new medical recruit swore by Apollo, Aesculapius, Hygeia and Panacea "to help the sick according to my ability and judgment, but never with a view to injury and wrongdoing . . . to give no deadly medicine to anyone if asked, nor suggest any such counsel . . . to abstain from every voluntary act of mischief and corruption, and from the seduction of females or males, of freemen or slaves . . . and not to divulge anything seen or heard in the course of professional practice."

Practising physicians were given advice on how to conduct themselves, which in an indirect way criticised the many who undoubtedly failed to live up to this standard; the following advice is a model to all who value the practice of this noble art:

"The doctor should know how to be silent at the proper moment and should conduct a regular life, because this contributes much to his good reputation. His behaviour should be that of an honest man and as such he should appear gentle and tolerant before honest men."

On this ethical note we can leave Greek medicine, and while we pay tribute to the considerable advances made in rational clinical medicine and in the discussions of the philosophical schools, we nevertheless recognise that the basis of Greek medicine in a slave society contained an innate weakness, particularly in the treatment of the downtrodden and the poor, which led on the one hand to an undue emphasis on religion and magical practices, and on the other to a contempt by the philosophers and the theoreticians for practice.

Chapter Four

ROMAN MEDICINE

The Empire Builders

WHILE the Greek culture was leisurely concerned with an ideal perfection far above the slave system on which it was based, there was developing in the Italian peninsula an irresistible force, driven by an ambition for conquest and wealth, which in the end overcame all the lesser Empires.

Where the slaves of Egypt and Greece had been numbered in thousands, those of Rome were counted in hundreds of thousands; where the Greek Empire was reaching the limits of the wealth it could extract from the output of its declining slave population, the Romans annexed new treasures in the course of their far-flung military adventures. The new Empire builders felt that they were acquiring untold wealth: they were, but again it was concentrated into the hands of a relatively small class. As with the Greeks, the Romans were content to use the cheap and plentiful slave labour as their main means of producing wealth, and the inner conflicts of the Greek Empire were intensified for the Romans, so that the collapse was on a much greater scale when it finally came.

Nevertheless, during its period of rising power, Rome met and overcame new difficulties on the road to civilisation which were victories more vital for humanity than those of empire-making.

In their constant drive for new territories for conquest and new markets for trade, the Romans generated a ferment amongst the peoples of their ever-expanding Empire, which gave birth to a rich internationalism in the exchange of commerce and of ideas.

From Britain to Ethiopia, from Russia to Morocco, from Iran to Spain, the streams of slaves poured towards the heart of the Empire, and among them were craftsmen and technicians, artists and medical men.

The Romans, like all conquerors, had much to learn from the conquered; they could count amongst their booty the special skills and knowledge of Greeks, Jews, Armenians, Germans, Negroes and Arabs.

On the other side of the world the Empire of China was also expanding, and about the first century B.C. the two great civilisations of the world again made contact, limited by the difficulties of communications, but at least some impressions of an exciting new world were gained by each: silks and perfumes from the East, potteries and bronze instruments from the West.

Foreign Doctors

The Romans were great road builders and law-makers; but in medicine they had to take their knowledge from the Greeks, even though they held them in contempt.

The total of Greek medical knowledge gained in centuries of strenuous study was concentrated in the great library established at Alexandria, the town built on the delta of the Nile by Alexander the Great. The Medical School at Alexandria continued for a time the true Hippocratic tradition of observation and research. Anatomy, physiology and experimental pathology were carried on; perhaps with too much enthusiasm, for, as recorded by Celsus, the Roman writer, "criminals were procured from prison by royal permission, and dissected alive". He added, "This was by far the best method of attaining knowledge".

A great effort was made by these Alexandrine doctors to discover the origins of disease, and they broke with the traditional idea of the four humours, and looked for causes in the local tissues and organs, a method of study which at least extended their knowledge of anatomy. Many notable advances were made in the understanding of the nervous system, and a clearer view was attained of the process of respiration, with the realisation that air was breathed in by the lungs.

Greek medicine had already collected valuable information on the use of herbs and drugs, and in this period of rival powers and fierce political jealousies, there was an added incentive to learn more about poisons and their antidotes. For the first time, opium was recommended, although with a warning that too much of it was dangerous; no doubt this drug was one of the more exotic importations from the new markets of the Far East. The medical men had a theory of prescribing gradually increasing doses of a poison in order to confer immunity against it—apparently the forerunner of modern methods of immunisation and vaccination. However, more indiscriminate prescribing was current, and it was carried to the absurd length of concocting a universal antidote incorporating over fifty ingredients, including viper's flesh. This type of hit-or-miss pharmacy has never failed in its popular appeal.

While Alexandrine medicine became one of the bridges that carried the best of the Greek medical tradition into Rome, its own standards declined with the decadence of the Empire. It became diverted from the broad principle of treating the patient and his environment as a whole, and adopted the concept of a local pathology; and soon there was a great number of specialists each treating an individual organ or a specific disease, with no thought for the patient as a complete person. The Alexandrine School of Medicine was finally lost in a confusion of mysticism, and religious and magical practices.

But life was intense and active in the Roman Empire, and to Rome came the foreign doctors who found poor employment at home; the city also attracted the charlatan, the self-seeker and the student. The three main schools of Greek medicine, the practical, the philosophical and the magico-mystical, established themselves in conditions which were similar to those in Greece; and each soon attracted its own following.

Medical science and public health had to find the answers to greater engineering and military problems than the Greeks had had to contend with, but as far as individual medicine was concerned, the Romans were handicapped by an even more pronounced contempt for the manual and practical arts, which they left entirely to slaves. The practice of medicine was considered merely another craft, essentially menial and fit only for slaves, many of Greek origin.

Roman senators and philosophers certainly had little confidence in doctors, particularly if they were foreigners. Cato wrote about them severely: "They have sworn to kill all barbarians with their drugs", and added significantly, "and they call us barbarians". Pliny the Elder wrote in a similar vein: "It is unfortunate that there is no law to punish ignorant physicians, and that capital punishment is never inflicted on them. Yet they learn by our suffering, and they experiment by putting us to death."

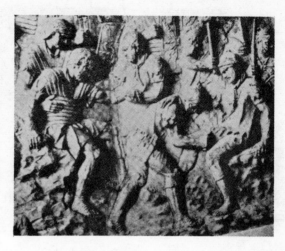

First-aid treatment in the Roman army.

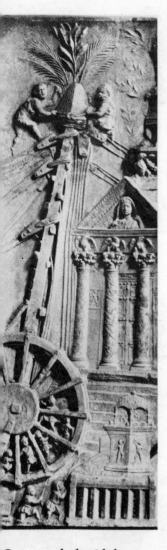

Crane worked with human treadmill.

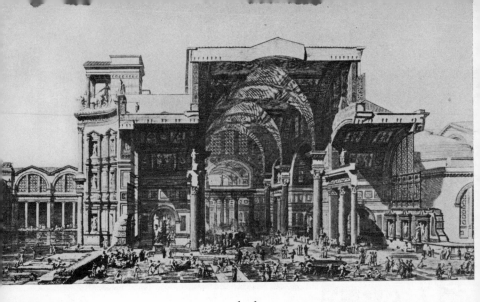

Roman baths.

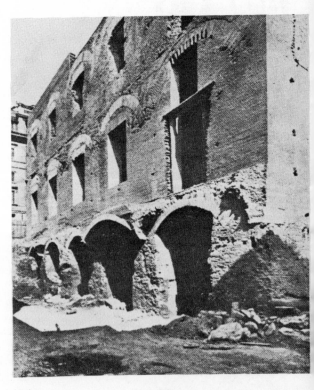

Street in Rome—Via Biberatica in Trajan's Market.

It is interesting to look at the comment about the Romans as barbarians, not from the standpoint of Cato, who considered this opinion simply as a sign of ignorance, but from that of the conquered Greek physicians, who came to this mighty capital only to find the old-fashioned superstitions about sickness still flourishing, while they had progressed so much further along the road of scientific healing.

In time, the Romans absorbed the Greeks' culture, but never equalled their achievements in medicine. They dealt rationally with the hygienic problems which obstructed their further advance as an empire-building nation: but, on the basis of their slave society, and with their infinite contempt for manual practice, they could not contribute much to original scientific thought. They were bound by shackles of their own making.

What the Roman Doctors Knew

Roman medicine, which had existed only in a primitive and unorganised way before the extension of the Empire, adopted the Greek methods of observation, but was always reluctant to come to close quarters with the everyday practice of the healing art.

More facts, however, were added to man's store of knowledge about sickness. Pneumonia, pleurisy, tetanus, diabetes, diphtheria, heart disease and tuberculosis were accurately described. Modern readers will recognise the "tuberculosis-prone" as the Roman saw them, "pale and slender, with shoulder-blades like wings or folded doors, prominent throats, and narrow chests". Diabetes was depicted as "a liquefaction of the flesh and bones into urine". The Romans had some insight into the various forms of insanity, which was recognised as a general disease which affected the patient emotionally and intellectually. One of the laws ensured that madmen be given into the care of the nearest relative, and a Roman physician was a pioneer in the introduction of more humane treatment of the mad. He insisted that they should not be kept in darkness (as was customary), since hallucinations were not increased by light, and he introduced occupational therapy, giving the patients exercises to help the memory and hold the attention; he also prescribed soothing music and wine to encourage sleep.

Like the Greeks, Roman practitioners gave serious thought to prognosis. They considered as bad signs feverish sweat and general fatigue, and any sudden increase or decrease in weight. They carefully examined the sputum, and in patients suffering from serious illness they recognised severe diarrhoea as a sign of approaching death.

So far so good: but the patient was most concerned with receiving the best treatment to aid recovery, and in this direction the Romans made no great headway.

The old Greek method based on establishing the even balance between the "four humours" was persisted in, with all the familiar "nature-cure" features: diet, massage, exercise and hydrotherapy. Moderation in all things was prescribed, and no doubt the richer-class Romans needed to be reminded to avoid excess in eating, drinking, excitement and sexual activities. Blood-letting, purgatives and emetics were popular forms of treatment; and also they had their slimming cults which recommended one meal a day, massage, exercises and less sleep. Sea voyages and a rest in the country were considered aids to recovery. It is clear what class of patients the doctors had in mind for this treatment; certainly, it was not intended for the poor or slaves.

Some ailments were dealt with very sensibly; for kidney diseases, suitable drinks which helped to cleanse the kidneys, hot baths, and the strict prohibition of salty and stimulating foods; for pneumonia, a light diet and frequent change of compresses and plenty of fresh air; and for diarrhoea, fasting followed by astringent food and drugs.

The Romans classified drugs according to the effects they produced, and there were four main divisions: purgatives, diuretics (acting on the kidneys), narcotics and emetics. This was a logical arrangement for doctors who tended to treat disease as though only one part or organ was affected, forgetting the wisdom of Hippocrates who saw the patient as a suffering human being in his individual environment. Different combinations of drugs were often prescribed, but some herbs were thought to have specific curative properties; for example, pepper for malaria, and parsley and celery for diseases of the kidney: these at least could do no harm.

One notable school of thought in Rome repudiated the "leave it to nature" attitude and thought that disease should be treated "speedily, safely and agreeably", although their methods did not differ very much from those of the nature-curers. They were guided, however, by a peculiar theory which was applied in all conditions; it simply postulated that good health depended on the state of the pores of the body. When these were too contracted or too relaxed ill-health followed. The cures which resulted from rational and practical treatment were ascribed by these doctors to their universal theory, which roused the enthusiasm of many citizens who were always ready to accept even a superficial panacea for their troubles.

New Facts and False Conclusions

The Romans accepted the practical methods of treatment from the Greeks, and like them, they suffered from a lack of knowledge of the body. They were soon to extend their experience, however, in the greatly enlarged field of military surgery and medicine, and as they became masters of great cities with ever-increasing populations, their medical knowledge grew in the department of public health.

They tried in a practical way to satisfy their curiosity about the workings of the living body by dissecting living creatures, such as monkeys and pigs. Methodically they investigated the body's structure. These were the nerves, this was how muscles worked; here was a difference between arteries and veins. They saw blood pulsing in the arteries, and took medical science one stride nearer the complete answer to one of its greatest queries, how the blood moved in the body. The Romans concluded wrongly that it must ebb and flow, and many centuries passed before medical knowledge arrived at a more complete picture of the circulation of the blood.

They carried out intelligent experiments on the animal body; for example, by damaging the brain and cutting the spinal cord, and studying the resultant forms of paralysis, they began to explore seriously the functions of the central nervous system. However, these dissections were too limited in scope to lead to any substantial advance in knowledge, and although they were well and accurately carried out, the Romans were misled by applying their new knowledge about animals to man, without modification.

The practical work, although realistic and useful, was made to fit itself into the old-fashioned cloak of the Greek philosophical school, which enveloped everything in a mysticism of magic numbers and migrating souls. The Romans followed uncritically the Aristotlean theme of searching for the divine perfection in all things, and many of their investigations into the functions of the body were guided by this sterile aim. The Romans, like the Greeks, raised their intellectual activities as far above practical work as masters were esteemed to be above slaves; the theories about divine purpose and pattern were therefore never put to the test of experience. The less these views were given a real test, the more dogmatic and prejudiced became their exponents. In the next 1,000 years this attitude grew completely hidebound and became impenetrable to any shaft of original thought.

The Roman doctors had learnt more about the workings of the body, and now they had to expound theories on their observations. Their efforts to keep in accord with the philosophy they had accepted produced some extraordinary views. Starting with the idea of a soul which had only a passing acquaintance with the body, they logically assumed a general world spirit, part of which was drawn into the lungs with the air man breathed. Other spirits controlled other parts of the body: natural spirits determining growth and nutrition through the liver; animal spirits activating the brain, and vital spirits (the essence of life) working through the heart. The various spirits moved in an ordered way through the veins and arteries; blood was supposed to flow from the chamber of the right side of the heart to one on the left, passing through (imagined) invisible pores.

As the constitution of the body was so imbued with intangible spirits, it followed that ill-health was accompanied by unpleasant changes in the different spirits, which upset the patient and his equilibrium. By a combination of this theory and the earlier Greek view of the four elements and humours in the body, the Romans produced a highly-coloured explanation of disease; fevers were said to be ephemeral in the spirits, putrid in the humours or fiery in the solids. Continued fevers, according to their duration, were either in the blood, the yellow bile, the black bile or the phlegm. One of the most serious errors was their belief that the pus which formed in wounds served a useful purpose, and they actually called it "laudable pus". They also read into the dreams of the patient a sign that the treatment was due for a change; in these matters they showed a duller clinical sense than the Greeks had done before them.

The Greek theory of curing by "opposite" was connected with the view that all illness was a condition of the body being either too relaxed or too rigid, and treatment was given accordingly. Purgatives and emetics were given for high blood-pressure or an overheated body; and if cold was supposed to have caused the sickness, heat was applied. Violent exercise was sometimes prescribed for the weak and sickly, a treatment which recalls the Spartan aim of kill or cure.

The Romans continued the intriguing occupation of making up drugs and potions which had been started in the earliest days when doctors were recognised as being primarily "medicine-men". The Romans worked scientifically, experimenting and learning from the reactions produced on the organism by the medicine, rather than by its colour, smell and taste.

They established methods of extracting, mixing and combining drugs which remained in use for the next 1,500 years. Claudius Galen, who lived about 100 B.C., and was an outstanding figure in Roman medicine, devised practical and valuable formulae which included such drugs as opium and hellebore. Cosmetic firms who produce such enormous varieties of goods today are frequently using the basic formula for cold cream, composed of oils, wax and rose water, which Galen prepared for beauty treatment nearly 2,000 years ago. Modern pharmacists also use simple vegetable compounds named galenicals after their creator.

The theory behind the practice, however, was not so admirable. Since Pythagoras' magic figure of four still dominated Roman philosophy, drugs, like everything else, contained this formula, and so they were composed of the four universal elements, fire, water, earth and air, and they shared the four qualities, hot, cold, moist and dry. This produced some strange reasoning about the innate qualities of drugs, but fortunately theorising was performed at a different level from the practical work, which progressed as long as it was unhindered by false thinking.

Roman Surgery

Man learns readily from experience, especially if he has efficient tools. In the field of surgery, the Romans had both. There were always surgical cases requiring attention, for Romans were engaged in continuous wars; and if not active in foreign wars, they had always the mock battle-field at home where gladiators warred with each other for the amusement of the populace.

The variety of wounds and injuries so incurred called for highly specialised instruments, and with the wide application of iron, the manufacture of surgical instruments became an important craft. Celsus, in his treatise on medical knowledge, described more than 100 different instruments, including forceps, scalpels, amputation saws and trephines, syringes and probes, and a special instrument for removing pieces of bone after the delicate operation of trephining the skull. He also mentioned an ingenious instrument, an iron in the form of a letter V, to keep the ends of the wound apart when removing arrowheads.

Excavations at Pompeii have unearthed over 200 different medical instruments, most of them found together in what may have been a craftsman's premises, or perhaps a shop. It was customary to obtain medical supplies in this way, because, according to Galen, in one of his writings, "the best shop for buying ligatures is in the Via Sacra between the Temple of Rome and the Forum".

The Romans had taken a small step towards overcoming man's deep-rooted horror and religious fear of dissecting the human body; and by studying the bodies of executed criminals they added to their anatomical knowledge.

They were prepared to undertake serious operations which had never before been thought possible, such as amputation for gangrene, and even for chronic ulcers, tumours and deformities. The patients concerned would certainly have bled to death, had not the Romans discovered the technique of applying ligatures where the simple remedies of cold water and vinegar proved useless. A Greek surgeon, practising during the most successful period of Roman medicine, gives the first written account of the method (similar to that used today) of arresting bleeding by catching up the smaller blood vessels with hooks and twisting them many times in order to close them.

The Romans were adept at other surgical operations, and many of their descriptions have entered into the classics of medical knowledge, such as their method of crushing stones in the bladder, and curing hernias. They were masters of the art of plastic surgery, and could restore the renowned Roman nose after injury by using neighbouring parts of the face for the cure.

Abdominal injuries were tackled with confidence. The patient was placed on his back with the pelvis raised; the wound was enlarged and the intestines put back in their place. The damaged part was cut away with scissors, and the wound sewn up, carefully bringing together the flesh as well as the skin. The patient was probably made unconscious by stiff doses of alcohol.

Fractures were treated in the true Hippocratic tradition. The bone being set, the limb was fixed with splints and bandages containing wax and starch to make them rigid; and these were renewed after a few days when the swelling went down. Exercises were prescribed to get the limb back to normal use.

The eye is a precious and delicate organ, and credulous Romans must have suffered considerably at the hands of the charlatans who claimed to be "eye specialists", but the surgeons could successfully treat one common complaint, cataract of the eye, by methods which are similar to those used today, of extracting the lens by using a needle.

During Roman times, it became less of a hazard to bring a child into the world, and infinitely more pleasant for the baby than it had been in earlier days. The mother received some pre-natal attention, and the doctor studied her physical condition and noted the position of the unborn child. If it was considered necessary, the baby was carefully manipulated into a better position in the womb; and the Romans were prepared in an emergency to carry out the Caesarean operation, so-called because Julius Caesar himself was reputed to have been born with medical assistance in this way.

The new-born baby was welcomed with affection and handled sensibly and hygienically. His eyes were bathed, and for the first two days he was fed on boiled honey, and then breast-feeding was the rule. Roman children suffered from rickets and other childhood disorders, which are dealt with in some detail in the medical text-books of that time.

Like other peoples, the Romans paid for their over-civilised way of life by suffering from bad teeth; but they compensated by evolving a high standard of dentistry, and some examples of their dental bridge work have remained to prove their skill. According to Martial, a famous Roman satirical writer, they had even achieved that ultimate refinement, false teeth.

But it was not in the approach to individual medicine that the Romans excelled. The nature of the problems forced on them by their military expansion required organising ability on a large scale, and the Romans made their most lasting contribution to medicine in dealing with medical matters associated with administration, public health and sanitary law.

Public Health and the People

Relics of Roman buildings and cities still have the power to evoke in the modern mind a respectful appreciation of the tremendous administrative achievements they represent.

An adequate water supply to the towns was recognised by the Romans as a necessity for public health; a super-abundance was the mark of a civilised way of life. For the citizens of Rome they organised a never-ending flow of pure water amounting to many millions of gallons a day. This was brought by fourteen large aqueducts, which were partly underground for many miles, and partly constructed on arched supports which still stand today. Not only Rome, but all the main cities which were subject to Roman domination, were modernised in this way, and there are records of at least 200 aqueducts, including the famous ones at Nimes, in France, and Tarragona, in Spain.

These plentiful water supplies helped to adorn the gardens and squares of the fashionable areas with fountains and running water. The centres of social life were the magnificent public baths, constructed of marble and decorated with glorious frescoes of different coloured stones, illustrating the handsome nude bodies which resulted from the cult of personal hygiene and healthful exercise. These baths could accommodate from 1,000 to 3,000 people, and had steam-heated accommodation which was as popular as the regular bathing places. In Rome alone there were over 800 baths for the use of soldiers and the public.

The well-appointed homes of the rich had their own water brought in through lead pipes, and the poor citizens obtained their supply from the nearest public fountains. Many cities purified the water supply, removing gross impurities by filtering through porous stone or sand.

Rome also had a good drainage system, and its outlet into the River Tiber has survived for 2,500 years. The large houses had lavatories flushed with water and connected with the main sewers, but the general arrangement was to have latrines in the houses, with cesspits which had to be cleared regularly, or latrines in the streets where a small payment had to be made. Carts removed these accumulations outside the city walls, to be used on the fields as manure. The famous Roman outlet, the Cloaca Maxima, was used first for surface water, and later for the disposal of sewage. The underground passages were cleaned by slaves, whose personal health was apparently of little concern to the public health administrators.

A vivid picture of life in Roman times was preserved for the interest of historians by the sudden volcanic eruption which ended the busy provincial life of Pompeii just a few years before the Christian Era began.

The very wealthy few lived in sumptuous mansions graced with marble columns, the rooms built round a central court with beautiful mosaic paving and all the modern conveniences of the times, baths, indoor sanitation, and sometimes central heating through flues. The middle classes occupied many streets of similar but smaller houses, each with its terraced gardens and other amenities.

But for the great majority, the poor craftsmen and the ordinary citizen and his family, housing was as bad as the general standard of living. Many, though members of a great Empire, were driven by an unseen whip. The fear of starvation forced them to work until they dropped with exhaustion, creeping to their broken-down hovels in the narrow, twisted streets of the great cities. In the countryside, peasants lived as their ancestors had done, in huts with beaten earth floors and only a hole in the roof to let out the smoke from the fire, round which the family cooked and slept.

Similar differences existed between the classes in death as in life. In the interest of public health, the Romans had strict rules about burials, which at first were carried out beyond the walls of the city. As the population increased, cremation was made compulsory. The rich Romans were given an elaborate ceremonial, and their remains were stored in the dignified marble urns which lined the walls of the specially built Columbarium. The poor were often cremated together, and their ashes buried in a common pit.

The Romans, even more than the Greeks, required the services of specially appointed medical officers, each of whom was made responsible for his own district. The work of our own modern public health officers is in many ways modelled on the pattern set by the medical officer in Roman times. His daily routine consisted of testing the accuracy of weights and the quality of food for sale in the market; and he had the power to destroy any that was tainted. The constant flow of poor people requiring treatment had to be attended to, and there was the regular work of supervising the drainage system, seeing that the streets were cleansed, and preventing foul smells. All the time the medical officer and his assistants had to keep a watchful eye on public baths, brothels, taverns and the all-important water supply. He worked together with the city architect and engineer, who were concerned with house and town planning and sanitary works. A vital responsibility was the maintenance of the military health service.

Medical officers were State-employed, and the charge was passed on to the public by a special tax. The doctors had to achieve high qualifications, and were appointed by a public assembly, which impressed on them the great civic responsibilities with which they were entrusted. They were also allowed to practise medicine for wealthy patients, and in A.D. 533 the Justinian Code found it necessary to advise public medical officers that their duty was "to choose to do honest service for the poorest rather than be disgracefully subservient to the rich".

Working Conditions and Health

With such an abundance of slave labour, it did not occur to the Romans to consider how working conditions affected health. Slaves were a cheaper commodity for Romans than they had been in Egypt or Greece, and their value as human beings fell accordingly.

Many slaves worked in the open air, and were not bound to the relentless pressure of a machine system; but the utmost of their energy was forced from them. They toiled, in the mills and on the farms, chained together and driven by the whip. Flogging was a common punishment for minor crimes; or even worse, they were condemned to work in the mines, which was only a slower form of death than the alternative punishment of being thrown in sport to wild animals.

A Roman writer, Lucretius, wrote of the workers in the gold and silver mines: "Know ye not by sight or hearsay how they commonly perish in a short time and how all vital power fails those whom the hard compulsion of necessity confines in such employment."

The minor craftsmen and impoverished freedmen supplied the great army of labour necessary to make the tools and carry through the tremendous constructions essential for building the Empire. Those who were so employed were selling not only their labour but their health, often their lives.

A contemporary account of the effect of industrial work deserves the last word: "The base mechanic arts, so called, have a bad name; and, what is more, are held in ill-repute by civilised communities, and not unreasonably, seeing they are the ruin of the bodies of all concerned in them, workers and overseers alike, who are forced to remain in sitting positions and to hug the gloom, or else to crouch whole days confronting a furnace."

Epidemics

With all their elaborate concern for public cleanliness and hygiene, the Romans were helpless before the sudden depredations of epidemic diseases which spread misery and death among the population.

The masses, living crowded together, their health undermined by hard work, were easy victims of germs. Doctors had observed correctly that some diseases, such as tuberculosis and plague, could be passed on from one person to another, and as in the Eastern races, lepers were shunned as "unclean", although this may have had only a religious significance.

Public health measures, such as drainage of the swamps and marsh ground in and near Rome, helped to restrict the spread of the most common of all devastating diseases, malaria; but the doctors when faced with a serious epidemic could only fall back on wishful thinking and pray to the currently popular god or goddess. Nevertheless, there were thinkers who did draw near to guessing facts which only a microscope could reveal.

In 36 B.C., a Roman philosopher wrote: "In time of drought, the swamps generate small animals, so small that the eye cannot see them; through the nose and the mouth they enter the body and cause illnesses which are difficult to cure." And two generations later, in A.D. 55, a Roman physician wrote: "Under the influence of hot weather, the swamps give off noxious exhalations and produce animals armed with injurious stings which swoop down on us in extraordinarily thick-winged clouds; this is how we often contract maladies of a hidden nature of which the physicians themselves do not know the cause."

But these were individual voices: epidemics spread more or less unhindered in the unhealthy conditions which prevailed. Their terrible effects were recorded by Roman historians because they were events which were dangerous to the stability of the Empire.

After the eruption of Vesuvius, which destroyed the cities of Pompeii and Herculaneum, tens of thousands of people died every day from infection, and fifty years later a plague killed more than a million. Typhus, plague, smallpox and malaria continued to rage at intervals for the next 200 years, and while the wealthy could get some effective treatment or leave the danger areas, the slaves and poorer citizens had to suffer without protection all the ravages of such diseases. Lucretius, writing of the last great plague before the downfall of the Empire, described "shepherds and farm labourers delivered over to death by poverty and disease".

The health of the people became so bad, and their strength so weakened that they could not sow their fields or reap the harvest of their labours, and the very foundations of the Empire crumbled at the base.

Pioneers in Military and Hospital Service

Rome marched to power on the strength and efficiency of an excellent military machine. The leaders soon learned from experience that the most reliable soldier is the one whose welfare is looked after.

At first, however, there were no army surgeons, as this was an undignified occupation for a freeborn Roman. The soldiers were given bandages, and when wounded had to care for each other from their limited knowledge. It soon became an old army trick to avoid service by simulating sickness, commonly by causing an irritation to the skin or forcing up blood in the phlegm. Galen, speaking for the authorities, gave a strong warning to malingerers: "The ignorant imagine that it is impossible for the physician to distinguish between those who pretend and those who speak the truth." But the ignorant, driven by discomfort and lack of suitable attention, continued to malinger. One large group of soldiers serving under an unpopular leader bandaged each other and pretended to be wounded.

In time, the immigrant Greek doctors won an established and recognised place for themselves in the Roman cities, and many were officially appointed to look after the soldiers and practise surgery where necessary.

Then the Roman gift for organising found the opportunity and the most favourable means. A full-scale army medical service was developed, with as many as four physicians in charge of each section of 1,000 to 1,500 men. Except in extreme emergency, the doctors found it inconvenient to treat the wounded person on the battle-field; and they organised special sites which were set aside for their first-aid, the earliest recorded "sick bays".

These were soon expanded into well-equipped camp hospitals attached to the army and serving its needs when on the march. The Roman Army, however, was campaigning all over Europe, and in many places remained as an occupying force. Permanent hospitals were set up in these garrison towns, and their services were available to highly-placed civilians and their families as well as to the armed forces. One Roman hospital situated on the Rhine, and whose general plan it has been possible to reconstruct, compares favourably with a small modern hospital. The hospital could accommodate altogether 200 patients, and was planned to allow good ventilation, hygienic drainage and the usual first-class water supply. The central corridor had thirty-eight small wards leading off; its sensible and efficient construction suggests an equally efficient atmosphere enjoyed during its lifetime by patients and doctors.

The hospital service was extended by the Romans to treat the sick poor, athletes and gladiators. On the large estates sick bays were founded for the slaves, and it was in such places that slave-physicians gained their experience. Sometimes the lady of the house turned her hand to a little "doctoring", and in fact in Roman times some women acquired skill in medical practice, particularly in midwifery, for which they were considered most suitable.

In the early days of the Greek Empire, doctors practised from surgeries and clinics, and temples of healing served the purpose of residential sanatoria. In 291 B.C., the Romans established on an island in the Tiber a temple of Aesculapius, intended for the treatment of sick slaves, and although they were sent there to die rather than be cured, it was a step forward from the custom that allowed masters to leave sick slaves to die of exposure. A popular homely remedy for the ill slave was to feed him on cabbage, "and," said Cato, "if a slave is ill and cabbage does not cure him, then he should be got rid of, for it is bad economy to feed men who cannot work". To such unfortunates, the island hospital in the Tiber was at least a protection from the final act of cruelty; and later it gave shelter also to the sick poor.

From such an inauspicious beginning the Romans developed the idea of hospitals where people could obtain medical treatment; finally they built a number of clinics, infirmaries, hospitals and temples of Aesculapius in Rome.

Doctors and Philosophy

Roman medicine was at its best in the practical aspect; in public health, the advance of surgery, and the creation of a hospital system, it had surpassed all previous developments. It suffered, all the same, from the weaknesses it had inherited from its Greek tutors, being unsupported by any profound philosophy of medicine and encumbered with old-fashioned religious practices.

Celsus sums up the general attitude of the more thoughtful medical men towards the philosophers' pronouncements on disease. He says, "If reasoning from theory could have made them so, then philosophers would have become the greatest of medical practitioners." But, as he well knew, "they have words in plenty and no knowledge of healing at all". He was troubled by the fact that doctors used different methods of healing in places as important as Rome, Egypt and Gaul. How could one decide which was the correct method when they all produced the desired result? It is difficult enough, he points out, when we know the cause of the condition, such as in wounds or eye trouble; it would be even more complicated in the many cases where the cause is quite unknown. He then decides that practice can be the only sure guide. How did doctors with such different theories reach the correct results? Celsus says: "This has happened, because they deduced lines of healing, not from obscure causes, nor from the natural actions, concerning which different opinions were held, but from the experiences of what had previously succeeded."

No great advance in knowledge could be made on this exclusively practical approach, where the benefits of reason and theory tested in practice were so completely ignored.

Popular Medicine

Such was the attitude to medicine of the best doctors in Roman times. What went on in the usual day-to-day work of the general practitioners was a confused mixture of all the different schools of thought, the practical, the philosophical, and the magical, working blindly and empirically with all the different problems that life threw up.

Many of the Roman upper classes could hardly bring themselves to come into contact with the common run of practising physicians, and they showed more respect for their time-honoured religious rites, the herbal remedies, the votive objects set up in the temples, and their household gods, each presiding over a different disease.

The practising physicians adhered to old-fashioned methods, and showed little awareness of the philosophical arguments which were being so hotly debated far above their heads. The most popular treatment required of the early Greek doctors in the Roman Empire were ointments for gladiators, love philtres for women of easy virtue, and blood-letting for slaves. Inevitably, this profitable field attracted a large number of charlatans and quacks, all of whom of course were self-styled "specialists". The Roman playwrights and commentators found much to satirise in these eccentricities. Cicero found the excessive number of specialists rather suspicious. "Do you suppose", he wrote, "that in the days of the Greek Hippocrates there were special physicians for diseases, others for wounds, and others again for the eyes?" This was a reasonable criticism in a time when medical knowledge was so limited that it could not well cover so many branches of knowledge at a specialist level.

Martial ridiculed the quack physicians who "cauterise ingrowing eyelashes, cure a relaxed throat without cutting, remove brand-marks from slaves, and 'cure' ruptures". Eye-troubles were very common and the oculists come in for a particular railing, as in his savage attack addressed to Quintus, an eye-specialist: "The blear-eyed Hulas would have paid you sixpence, O Quintus. One eye is gone, but he will still pay threepence; make haste and take it, brief is your chance; when he is blind, he will pay you nothing."

Doctors still clung to supernatural beliefs when all else failed. The temples were always full of people praying for protection. There were goddesses to protect virgins or help pregnant women to have an easy delivery, and there were gods and goddesses to whom frantic prayers were offered in times of epidemics. The supreme god of health was the Greek god, Aesculapius, and his cult was followed in Rome with as much fervour as it had received in Greece.

Darkness over Rome

Rome's greatest hour had long passed; the vast gains made at the expense of other peoples had resulted only in economic and political crises as Rome's dependencies became greater and her power to create real wealth diminished.

In such times of stress, the wise men of Rome used their knowledge not to lead men out of darkness, but to take them even further backwards, and were blind to the fact that in mass ignorance they would all perish. We have already seen that Plato had advised that citizens should be taught "a noble lie", noble in so far as it was to help preserve the supremacy of the masters over the slaves; and Polybius, a great counsellor of Rome's decaying period, asserted that "the foundation of Roman greatness is superstition".

Rome's achievements had been great, but within her massive cities the enslaved people were growing ever poorer; the value of wages was falling, and more and more peasants were driven into the unproductive life of military service, their farms ruined and neglected.

When men came back from service, they had to face fierce competition in the labour market from the thousands of imported slaves who also had to work in order to live. The despised hand-manufacture of goods was more and more turned over to slaves; the demands of the home market grew smaller. Profits were not invested in industry, but in the more respectable channels of farming or money-lending, a growing profession to finance overseas trade. Industry was no longer expanding. Economic and political crises shook the stability of the Roman Empire and added the final blow to the results of the epidemic diseases and the deep-rooted social and moral unrest which was shattering the Empire from within.

Decadence was everywhere, permeating all the arts, the sciences, and the theory and practice of medicine. Religion offered an illusory avenue of escape to medical men, and for the next 1,000 years after the break-up of the Roman Empire, they trod this mystic path in philosophical medicine.

Chapter Five

THE MEDIEVAL AGE

Progress in a Dark Age

IF the history of man could be viewed as though from a great height, it would be seen to be in continuous movement, now and again breaking out into whirlpools of activity which in turn affect the stream of events which follow.

During violent historical changes much that was valuable to man can be lost; but new ways of living, a new search towards truth gathers momentum because what is imperishable in man is his urge to survive and be productive.

Egypt burned a sombre but steady light for many centuries; Greece flamed into brief brilliance, and Rome caught the reflected glory and shed it across the known world. Each in their turn were subdued by their own faults and a new force from outside. The barbarian hordes that swept down from the north upon the falling Roman Empire seemed to put out completely the light of Roman wisdom. The centuries that followed have become known as the Dark Ages, and this was by contrast with what had preceded and what came after.

The scientific and cultural achievements of the past endured, but some of the refinements of living were swiftly swept aside.

The barbarian conquerors had to continue ordinary daily life after the heat of battle had cooled. They had defeated a people, but they had not exterminated them. Trade and production had to continue, and the craftsmen, merchants, scientists and physicians were required to practise their arts and skill as in the past.

The New Age spread over Europe and the Mediterranean cities on the basis of an improved agricultural system, with a more powerful iron plough, heavily wheeled and drawn by horses, which was well suited to the wetter, richer soil of northern lands.

Many slaves had toiled with the slightest of tools in the ancient lands of the East. The great feudal landlords had no use for absolute subservience, but needed men who had some feeling of personal attachment to and interest in the soil which gave them all a living. The working people of this new age had not thrown off all the chains of slavery; they could still be sold by the lord of the manor as he sold his cattle. But they had gained some important rights; the farming implements were their property, and there was a small part of the land they could call their own and work in their own time.

The evolution of writing in the ancient world gave immortality to men's thoughts; with the invention of printing in the twelfth century A.D., this attribute gained wider significance. Hitherto, books had been laboriously copied by hand and libraries of manuscripts were too precious to be handled by the multitude.

The centre of civilisation had by now moved northward from the Mediterranean. Industry, agriculture and trade flourished in Northern Europe, and the population increased. And in the midst of all this ferment, doctors and physicians continued the practice and philosophy of an art whose roots spread far backwards to very different times.

The Church Thinks for the People

The Germanic and other barbarians who had overrun Rome had held primitive and bloodthirsty religious beliefs; their medical practices were mixed up with sacrificial rites, and the devils and demons who caused ill health were exorcised with herbs like mandragora, verbena and sage. Drinks made from mistletoe were believed to have a favourable effect on infertile women; our Christmas custom of a kiss under the mistletoe has a long history.

These superstition-ridden barbarians were able to impose a new social structure on the decayed slave empire, but the more advanced philosophy and unified religious force of Christian Rome exerted a domination which finally expressed itself in the unassailable power of the Church.

The Church developed its might step by step with the other rulers of the people, the kings, the lords and the barons. It preached a dogma which restated in terms of its own era the orthodox view of all previous régimes, namely, that the masses should look for their delivery from sorrow only in the life after death.

Being of such support to the rulers of the time, the Church gained a privileged share in the lands and the increasing wealth. The great achievements of the medieval Church were its preservation of the written knowledge of Greece and Rome, and its creation of centres of culture in all parts of Europe where cathedrals were raised to the glory of God and thousands of anonymous craftsmen.

Much earnest effort went into copying the classical scientific and literary texts, but the religious brothers seemed to be concerned with the artistic effect of their writing, rather than with the meaning of the thoughts they were transcribing. The rigid Church dogma glossed over and distorted the free-thinking philosophy of the Greeks, but it was important that some of that knowledge was being preserved for rediscovery in the future.

Besides the technique of fine writing, the Church encouraged other arts which centred round the remarkable cathedrals, stained-glass windows, fine tapestries, carvings and stone sculpture; mechanical clocks with fascinating moving figures enthralled the worshippers of the thirteenth century, as they still captivate the sightseers today in Prague, Venice, Wells and York.

The suffocating dogmatism of the early Christian Church was dispelled to some extent by a fresh breeze of knowledge spreading from Iran in the sixth century and from Arabia from the eighth to the tenth centuries. The Arabian conquests unified further areas of the inhabited world, and a different intellectual approach to man's view of the world encouraged a greater tolerance of conflicting opinions. Nevertheless, the Church had by now deeply established itself both for Heaven and on earth; with all its authority it maintained that Heaven would confer eternal happiness, to which the peasant and serf could aspire only by dutifully accepting without protest their appointed place on earth.

Despite the Church teaching, conditions for the people frequently became too hard to bear, and under Wat Tyler in the fourteenth century, English serfs asserted by open revolt the right of men to live as men and not as slaves or beasts. The Hussite wars in Bohemia and the Peasant War in Germany in the sixteenth century continued the living link in this long struggle for human dignity, which stretched backwards across the ruins of Rome, Greece and Egypt.

Faith and Healing

The old beliefs die hard. Even while the Christian Church was establishing its superiority over other forms of religion, the temples of Aesculapius were still producing their miracles of healing, and so winning the worship of yet more pagans.

The Church could not tolerate such rivalry, which affected people in their most vulnerable emotion, the fear of disease and death. What the Word could not subdue was overcome by the Sword. The pagan temples were overthrown and the medical divinities removed from their shrine in the thoughts of the people. However, the longing for release from pain, and the faith in mystic methods, could not be so easily wiped out of men's minds. The Church simply took over the whole ritual, making it an essential part of the practising religion of the day: so the models of healed limbs which had been pagan offerings were dedicated to the Church; and to the Church the patient went, to sleep the sleep of the faithful, receiving the dream oracle and cure in the name of a new Divinity which superseded all others.

The influence of religious beliefs, therefore, strongly determined the evolution of new medical theories and practice from the West to the East. Christian teaching emphasised the earlier belief that sickness and disease were punishments that fell on man for his sins. There was nothing he could do about this but atone by fasting and prayers. Against this dogmatism, the rational clinical teaching of Hippocratic medicine was ineffective; in fact, a rational approach to ill health was considered sacrilegious and a direct criticism of the Great Physician, God. The human body, being a divine creation, could not be subjected to the impious hands of dissectors, and so its study at first hand was condemned as a crime against God and man.

The Christian attitude to medicine at that time reverted to the views held by men at their most primitive. Augustine epitomised it in his dictum. "All diseases are to be ascribed to Demons." Such a bigoted view encouraged the wildest forms of irrational treatment. Instead of the incantations of the old Egyptian priests, recitals of the Creed or Paternosters were made over the patient; primitive charms and magical formulae were given a medieval dress, but the foundation was the same. Monks and clerics were forbidden to practise medicine, and so in time the Church severed its connection with progressive scientific thought, which lived on in spite of all religious proscriptions.

The church dignitaries themselves were not free from the continuous conflicts between their beliefs and their understanding. There is a story of a cleric who treated his toothache by touching his cheek with a holy curtain hanging from the shrine of a saint; but he also called in the aid of a surgeon. He then suffered a worse torment than toothache, and was driven to confess that "by a suggestion of the Enemy" he could not escape the thought that the surgeon alone might have achieved the cure.

The Church tried to condemn magico-mystical forms of medical treatment, but its resistance to rational medicine eased the way for all forms of charlatanism. It established the superiority of the belief in one God to the polytheism of pagan times, but as the Church still considered disease to be a punishment of divine origin, people expected a corresponding mysticism in treatment.

As royalty was the expression of Divinity on earth, it was logical that the ancient belief in the power of the king's touch should be revived; and in England, Edward the Confessor had the dubious pleasure of laying hands on scores of his subjects suffering from scrofula, the skin disease known then as "the King's evil"; and this custom continued until the days of Queen Anne.

The old incantations experienced a new popularity; they were freely translated into the idiom of the day, and taken quite seriously. It was common knowledge that if a man's nose bled, he could be cured by whispering in his ear on the same side "at least thrice nine times—'socsocam sykyma'—and you may go on saying it". No doubt the nose-bleed ceased before the healer grew tired. If a person with an aching tooth was lucky enough to suffer on a Tuesday or a Thursday, and when the moon was waning, it was possible to effect a cure by saying "argidum margidum stargidum" seven times.

There is an echo of the ancient Egyptian practice in the preparation of an ointment, which had to be mixed to the continuous intonation of the words: "The God of Abraham, the God of Isaac, and the God of Jacob, give virtue to this salve."

Such medical treatment was not entirely irrational; incantations were often merely an accompaniment to the practical side; for example, in removing a bone stuck in the throat, it was considered a help to cry out during the operation: "As Jesus Christ drew Lazarus from the tomb, and Jonah from the Whale, thus Blasius, the martyr and servant of Christ, commands: 'Bone come up or go down'."

Precious stones were considered to have healing properties, just as had the amulets of old, and were worn as prevention; which was no more irrational than the contemporary custom of wearing a camphor bag on the chest to ward off colds or iodine lockets to guard against rheumatism.

Naturally, the charlatans had great scope for their histrionic abilities, but they were not without insight, as can be seen from the medieval practitioner who gave advice on impressing the patient by telling him that he is suffering from obstruction of the liver. "Be sure to use the word 'obstruction'", he writes, "for they don't understand it, and it is often exceedingly useful that people should not understand what you say."

Cleanliness, Godliness and Christian Charity

The influence of Christian thought, at least in the Middle Ages, did little to spread the idea that cleanliness was next to Godliness; in fact, if this life had meaning only as a spiritual preparation for the next, the less people regarded the daily creature comforts the better for their souls. However, the hope that good deeds on earth would most surely win heavenly reward, encouraged the practice of Christian charity. Some of the teachings of Jesus which had been inspired by sympathy with the downtrodden and the persecuted were interpreted by the Church as a religious duty to succour the sick, the helpless, the orphan and the homeless.

Money was collected from the faithful and the fearful, and the Church established almshouses and orphanages where the outcasts and shattered wrecks of a ruthless world could find some small security and medical care. These beneficiaries of charity were in no danger of being pampered. The sick were nursed by clergy or widows attached to the Church, who were untrained. Half the orphans who came under the charitable roof did not survive the unloving care they received; the remainder were soon sent out into the world to find what employment they could as farm workers or in menial positions in one or other of the town guilds of craftsmen.

The Church, however, had established the important principle that authority must assume some responsibility for those in need. If all men could not be treated as brothers, ignoring the Christian maxim, society at least could not deny the urgent claims of its poorest relations.

With medical and sanitary knowledge so restricted, the problem was indeed vast; but cities and lands were accumulating wealth and resources. Early in the ninth century, Italian cities accepted as a civic duty the protection of children, lunatics, the blind, the deaf and the dumb, and special institutions were established for their care. By the thirteenth century Belgium had a relieving office in every parish which helped with money or gifts to those in desperate need. Most European countries had similar problems and dealt with them with the beginnings of a social conscience.

Hospitals in the Making

The example of the Church in setting up institutions to help the sick poor was followed by the brotherhood of monks, who lived and worked in monasteries closely associated with the Church. Monks withdrew from a world that seemed to them to be evil, and they hoped by prayer and fasting to save not only themselves but all men.

They lived together in small communities, acquiring land and other valuable possessions which called for attention and industry; they soon departed from their early vows of poverty and stoicism. Some monasteries emerged as self-contained villages, with bakehouses, breweries, stables and barns, and a variety of craftsmen with well-equipped workshops. Beside the picture of the lean, ascetic monk, there is the equally authentic one of the "jolly friar", frequently rather too jolly, so that a custom was established in the monasteries to bleed the brothers at regular intervals to protect their health from the ill effects of too much eating, and drinking of ale and wine.

The monasteries were soundly built and well-drained, with good water supplies. The monks themselves were not of particularly pleasant habits, and many, like their less pious fellows, rarely washed and were vermin-ridden. However, the monasteries advanced simple rules of hygiene which no doubt the monks had been forced to recognise, living in such proximity with each other.

It was counselled that although the body need be washed only two to three times a year, the feet should be washed once a week; certainly a great advance on no washing at all. The monk also received instruction in table-manners; he "was not to cast forth upon the table the superfluity of fish or other meat, not to crack nuts with his teeth for another guest, not to cough or sneeze without turning away from the table, not to wipe hands or teeth on the cloth".

The monks were expert agriculturists, and expanded their wealth by the industrious cultivation of the land, by fruit growing and by sheep farming. They were not unlearned, and many monasteries established libraries and schools which were the foundation of secular education. But by removing themselves from the ordinary run of their fellow-men, they could not in fact uproot themselves from the earth on which all live. They had more time to observe events and people, and they eventually became the historians of their day, leaving records and chronicles of great value.

However, the most socially useful activity of this well-intentioned brotherhood was the open house which they kept for travellers of all types, from the homesick soldier to the refugee from pestilence or other terrors. Benevolent hospitality meant that the monasteries or the houses of the bishops should set apart some rooms for the comfort of the weary pilgrim; food there was in plenty. But during the time of the Crusades, a greater strain was thrown on the charity of the monks by the plight of large numbers of soldiers, war refugees and sick people in dire need of shelter and help.

Throughout Western Europe infirmaries were established, usually attached to monasteries. Some of these were well-equipped with separate wards for the mild and serious cases, but many had simple straw mattresses only, and medical care was elementary. However, the patient was given food, warmth and kindness, and religious services which soothed even if they could not cure.

These infirmaries were the beginnings of the present-day hospital service. A typical thirteenth-century hospital was the Hotel-Dieu in Paris, which had four wards and a staff of about sixty drawn from the religious brotherhood and sisterhood, with four priests at the head.

The conditions of the patients would horrify the modern nursing school, but the monks saw nothing dangerous to health in crowding the sick people naked, two to a bed, and with scarcely room enough to pass between the beds. Everything was performed in the ward, from operations to laying out the dead; inevitably, spreading infection and gangrene were common, and the only known remedy was to spray the wards several times a day to mask the terrible smell. The "madmen" among the sick—and there must have been many—were bound and confined in special cots.

The familiar names of many London hospitals honour the far-off founders of what have been permanent institutions for hundreds of years. St Bartholomew's (1123) and St Thomas's (1215) were named by the pious monks who attended the sick poor of London under these medieval roofs.

From the beginning the demands made on the hospitals were greater than their resources. To help the good work, inmates of the hospitals were forced to beg alms in the streets, and in some towns a charge was put on the local rates. The mayor and local officials inspected the premises from time to time.

The work which had begun through the charitable impulse of the monks laid deep foundations in the organised life of the people. In the time of Henry VIII, the power and influence of the monasteries was broken and the noble order of nursing was established on a secular basis. Nursing societies were organised which took no religious or perpetual vows, as did the nursing sisters of the Church. These societies grew, particularly in Continental countries such as Germany, France and Sweden.

Lords and Serfs

The literary and artistic pictures that have been drawn of the Middle Ages give an impression of great bustle and activity and of vivid contrasts which, if studied in detail, show that the Middle Ages were continuing the tradition of the rich man in his mansion, the poor man in his hut. Since the general population was poor, there was no great change for most people in their share of overcrowding, dirt and poor feeding, and therefore no end to the sorry tale of spreading epidemics and infections which continuously afflicted the population, often affecting the rich as well as the poor.

In the country, the lord of the manor enjoyed every comfort and luxury that wealth could buy and that the working people could produce for his delight. To "live like a lord in his manor" was to live as well as any millionaire can do today, making allowances for the limited production of the period. To live like a peasant family was to share a one-roomed hut, smoky and draughty, dark and cold in the winter and stifling in the summer. During the winter most of the rural inhabitants found warmth, comfort and conviviality at the local inn, or even at the smithy. It was cheering, but scarcely the healthiest way of spending the few leisure hours left after exhausting work in the fields and on the farms.

Town life for the masses was even more squalid. The people lived in "quaint" little houses which were dark, damp and grossly over-crowded. Down the middle of the narrow, unpaved street an open drain received all the garbage and excrement, sometimes carelessly thrown out of the overhanging upper stories; neither sunlight nor fresh air could penetrate the putrid atmosphere.

The nearest attempt at town planning directed certain offensive trades to move beyond the city walls or to keep to their own streets; so that today in London we have a memory of these times in "Butchers' Row", and "Tanners' Lane"; and the Continental evil of confining the Jewish population within a well-marked ghetto was copied in England. Burials were unregulated, and the dead were crowded together with no regard for the hygiene of the living.

The water supply to London was conveyed recklessly along open channels, which were often used as a convenient dumping ground for rubbish. Londoners bought their supply from water-carriers, with no guarantee asked or given for its purity. To add to the general unpleasantness, the public latrines were never flushed; even the large houses, who at least had their private cesspools, rarely had them emptied.

The people lived in these hovels with less comfort than the domestic animals who often shared their roof. Families slept two by two in uncomfortable bunks, without bedclothes or night-wear. The small windows had only canvas or waxed cloth stretched across the opening; and in these unlovely rooms, promiscuity, venereal disease and infection spread like the vermin that infested the dark corners.

The houses were mostly timbered, with roofs thatched with reed or rush; in the small towns the people were not completely excluded from the native beauty of orchards and gardens which surrounded the cottages, often with space for poultry yards, cow byres and stables. But this fragment of comfort was doomed in time to be devoured by the hungry growth of the industrial town.

As they lived, so they ate. The solid oak banqueting tables of the nobility were laden daily with every kind of meat and game, with rare fruits such as pomegranates and oranges imported from Spain, and with wines from France, Spain and Italy. The wife of a nobleman in any part of medieval Europe had to be skilled in the art of administering a large household run by dozens of servants, all revolving round the comfort of the family. The master of the house did not qualify as a gentleman until he had learned how to carve correctly the many luxurious meats which he and his guests enjoyed, often with the added pleasure of music and entertainment.

The lower classes required no special training to serve the coarse brown or black bread made of rye or a mixture of rye and wheat which was their daily food. The very poorest had to live on a substitute made of pea or bean flour, and very little else.

Besides bread, the workers ate fish in every condition, except fresh and wholesome: it was salted, pickled or dried; but salt was dear, and the fish was often putrid. Ale was a popular drink which helped to keep their spirits high; water was the last resort of the very poor.

Some effort was made to improve the quality of the food sold. Fines were imposed for adulteration or contamination, but the traders found (as some traders always will until the fines exceed the profit) that it was worth while to pay up and continue their onslaught on the public purse and health. Sometimes the fines were computed on a yearly basis, so the civic conscience was salved.

The widespread underfeeding and poor standards of health and hygiene provided a fruitful breeding-ground for all the infectious diseases that made the face of the Middle Ages appear pockmarked and disfigured to later generations.

The working conditions of the people added the final blot to this

picture of stunted and deformed humanity. Workers had no protection from the risks of industries, where they toiled in winter from
dawn to dusk, and in summer from four in the morning until eight
at night; there was a half-hour rest for breakfast, and later another
break for about an hour and a half, to enable them to pause and
recover breath enough to complete the day's labour.

The many artistic and architectural achievements of medieval times
were created by workers suffering from new industrial diseases, including lead poisoning contracted in preparing paint and mining
lead; tuberculosis promoted by dust breathed while cutting stone
statuettes and images; and mercury poisoning which afflicted the
craftsmen who in the course of their elaborate gilding work, had to
heat the amalgam to drive off the mercury, much of which was
absorbed by their own bodies.

The Price the People Paid

No society can avoid the consequences of its way of living. Man
has suffered through the ages from ailments of which we still do not
know the cause, such as diabetes, stone in the bladder and different
forms of rupture, but he has also made the conditions which encouraged diseases, such as famine pestilences, plague and smallpox,
afflicting hundreds of thousands.

The survivors of these frequent epidemics were left in their unhealthy tenements, weak in body, and ready victims for new squad-
rons of germs bringing dysentery, consumption, boils and many
forms of fever to the battleground. The people of the dark ages had
no medical defences against these attacks. In addition they were pecu-
liarly subject to such debilitating ailments as palsies, St Vitus's dance,
and hysterical forms of illness, very common among women, which
doubtless had their origins in the fearful superstitions which took the
place of a rational philosophy in their minds.

Their food was not only of poor quality, but was frequently the
cause of specific troubles, such as ergotism, a disease which was widespread in France because bread was often made of infested rye; in
Northern Italy, where maize was the main constituent of the diet,
a deficiency of vitamins produced physical distress and premature
death among the peasants.

Because of the low standards of life and the endless working day, the economic development of Europe was often held back by great waves of illness overtaking the working population.

We are coming now to the beginning of Britain's recorded history, and from the Anglo-Saxon Chronicles and other records, we learn that about fifty epidemics attacked Britain from the end of the seventh century to the beginning of the fourteenth. The descriptions do not give exact details of the infections, but it is apparent that they included typhoid, smallpox, diphtheria, tuberculosis, and, without question, the plague.

The Black Death

"The Dark Ages" have become almost synonymous in people's minds with "The Black Death", so great an impact did this scourge make; for at the time of its greatest spread, it must have seemed to the civilised world that, after all the victories over nature, mankind was to be annihilated by this terrible disease.

The great sea-routes which had brought goods from the ports of Asia and Europe, now brought from as far as China an unwanted cargo, which none could reject. Sometimes ships drifted aimlessly, every man on board stricken down by the same black hand of death.

The rich in the large towns fled to the country, closed their doors and their ears to the devastation outside, and recounted fairy stories to pass the time and forget their fears. In this way the famous *Decameron* of Boccaccio was written, but in the preface the author writes of the terrible reality from which he was helping his rich patrons to escape. He tells how medical treatment was powerless to halt the illness, which often ended in death within three days.

Infection seemed to lurk in every corner. Even coming in contact with an animal which had belonged to a sick or dead person was enough; to speak to a sufferer, or to handle anything he touched, was to invite disaster. It was bad enough for the rich, who had to leave their usual comforts and even so run the uncertainty of having been infected; but for the rest of the population it was much worse; Boccaccio tells their pitiful story:

"The case of the poor, and perhaps most of the middling, was far more wretched; for most of these men were kept at home either by hope or by poverty, and in those close quarters, they sickened daily by thousands and, for lack of service and all else, almost all were irrevocably doomed to death. Many breathed their last in the open streets by day or night; many again, though they ended in their own dwellings, gave the first notice of death to their neighbours by the stench of their rotting corpses; and whether in this fashion or in that, death reigned everywhere. . . . Nor were the country districts spared; for throughout our scattered villages and homesteads the wretched labourers and poor folk, with their families, died without any help of physician or succour of servants, breathing their last by the roadside or among the crops, or in their cottages, by day and by night alike, not like men, but almost like beasts."

Boccaccio describes how in this "end of the world" atmosphere, chaos came upon the orderly government of affairs. The guardians of the laws were themselves afflicted, and too far involved in personal tragedy to consider the general welfare.

There is a graphic description written by a contemporary doctor who had clearly tried to grapple with the disease, but he was forced to share the general despair. He wrote:

"A burning pain, starting either in the groin, or under the armpits, gradually spread over the region of the heart, and the vital parts were attacked by a mortal fever. The heart and lungs were affected and the respiratory passages were choked with the poison. The strength suddenly declined and the patient could only survive a few days. There seemed no refuge from this scourge, neither heat nor cold, nor the fresh country air, the cold north or the warm south. So contagious was it that where sickness commenced in a house scarcely one escaped. The slightest contact, a single breath, sufficed to transmit the disease. Those who tried to aid the sick fell victims. The ill-nourished were easily stricken. Those who lived a temperate life fared best. The number of the dead was greater than the number of survivors, and cities were deserted, thousands of houses standing with open doors or locked up, their owners dead or fled."

This first experience of the plague was to be repeated every few years for the next three centuries, but never again with such a devastating effect; the last record of a widespread epidemic was the Great Plague in the seventeenth century, but by that time conditions had changed and medical knowledge had emerged from the low level to which it had fallen after the eclipse of Greek and Roman science.

Panic and Precautions

The view that diseases were "catching" had been held in Biblical times by the Jews, who introduced very strict laws of isolation in certain diseases. The Greeks classified tuberculosis, ophthalmia, plague and leprosy as contagious. From their own observation medieval physicians added to this list smallpox, pestilential fevers, and various forms of ulcers and skin ailments, including scabies. Their theories, however, did not match the shrewdness of their observation.

Some authorities held that the cause of the plague was due to the conjunction of Saturn, Jupiter and Mars on the astrologically ill-omened date of 24 March, 1345. Other theories suggested it was due to the poisoning of wells by lepers and Jews, or alternatively to the wrath of God for the sins of mankind; a more rational theory was that the infection emanated from corruption in the air, or issued from standing water and privies. The theorists on both sides of the university walls were bewildered. Learned professors of medicine contradicted the Greeks by maintaining that tuberculosis was hereditary; nevertheless, they borrowed the out-dated Greek theory of "the humours", and suggested that their maladjustment caused scabies. If professors went so far astray, it is not surprising that the ordinary medieval doctor was as much a victim of superstition as was the mere layman.

However, the knowledge that disease was spread by contact gave the authorities a guide to action, and gradually some precautionary measures were introduced.

The first task was to track down the danger spots from which infection spread. A law was passed that infectious cases must be notified, and penalties were imposed to counter a natural reluctance to become a voluntary outcast in this way. To enforce the law, the authorities employed "searchers" whose need for the payment was stronger than their panic. Carrying white wands, they searched the streets, marked infected houses with a sign, and barred doors and windows from the outside. The unfortunate inhabitants were virtually cut off from the world, and depended on the uncertain kindness

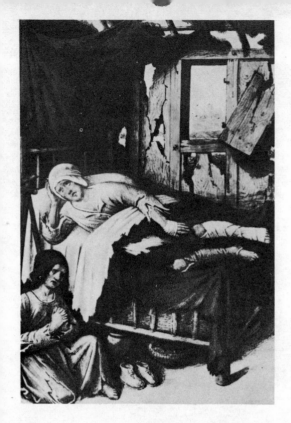

Village hovel—interior.

Reconstructed interior—fourteenth-century hall.

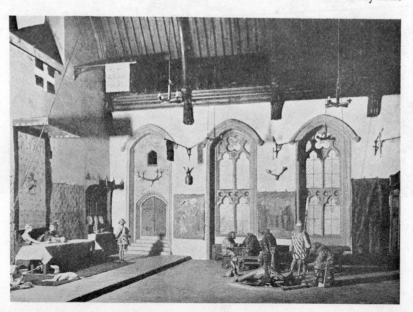

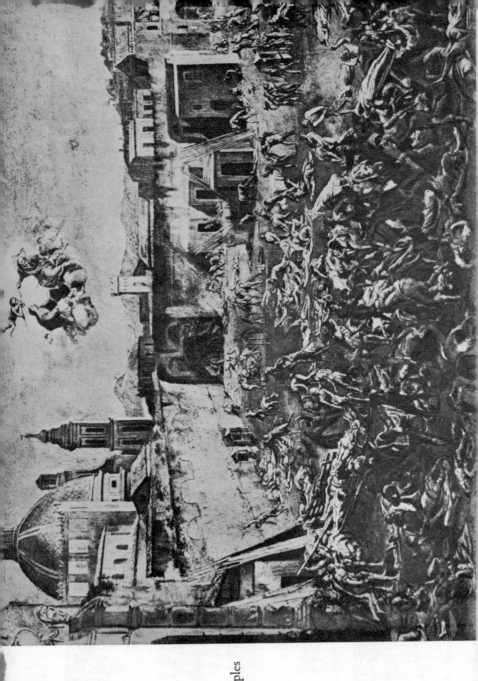

Plague scene, Naples
(1656).

of neighbours or relatives to thrust a little food or drink through the barred windows. Through the quickly emptying streets the searchers called on the bereaved to bring out their dead, so that they could carry off the corpses for hasty burial.

By the fifteenth century the law ordered that infected homes must "put out wisps and bear white rods", as a warning sign, and it was also forbidden to keep animals, whose movements could not be so easily controlled.

The results were encouraging. Law and order could, it was becoming clear, put some restraints even on the ever-smouldering threat of pestilence. The clues to follow were those that incriminated dirt as a source of infection. By the sixteenth century, it was a civic responsibility to see that lanes and streets were kept reasonably clean. Into the purifying fire went refuse, infected clothing and bedding. The house that showed a warning sign was kept closed for forty days.

The authorities threw their net wider. What about the nauseating slaughter-houses, with their welter of blood and slime? They had to come under control, and also the workplaces of bedding upholsterers, who used the most questionable and unhygienic materials. It was obvious that the responsibility for public hygiene could not be left to the initiative of private people, and from this time onwards, the local authority organised scavenging and sanitation. Another important improvement was the supervision of burial grounds; overcrowding was forbidden, thus showing some respect for the dead and consideration for the health of the living.

The authorities had taken to heart all the bitter lessons learnt from the first onslaught of the Black Death; they knew that in all probability it had been brought from across the seas, and special care was taken with ships and cargoes from abroad. These remained in open harbour until they had been exposed to the effect of sun and wind and they were then fumigated. If there was still some doubt, the goods were destroyed and the ships sent post-haste away. So it was with confidence that by the sixteenth century, Shakespeare could write:

> *This fortress built by Nature for herself*
> *Against infection and the hand of war . . .*

Other medieval townships were conducting a similar battle. The port of Venice had special sanitary inspectors to carry out the regulations on quarantine. As in England, travellers and homeless people suspected of plague were isolated in "pest-houses" placed outside the city. The Venetian authorities tried in many ways to prevent a recurrence of an epidemic. In times of danger, people were advised to take special diets, avoid bathing and sexual intercourse, and wash with vinegar, which was considered a useful disinfectant, perhaps because it causes a stinging sensation. It was also employed to wash gold, which was presumed to spread infection widely when passing from hand to hand. All things which came in contact with infected people were disinfected thoroughly; items of small value were burned, and bedding was set out in the sun to be purified; water that tasted or smelled offensively was boiled.

The physician of the Middle Ages adopted a special outfit designed to protect him as much as possible from contact with the patient. He was covered from head to foot in a dark, flowing gown, his hands and arms hidden inside long gloves; and from his hooded face there protruded a long beak containing protective perfumes and spices. This was the medieval doctor, and it makes one wonder who was more frightened of the other: the doctor or the patient. All the physician could do for the sufferer was to comfort him and spray the room with pleasant perfumes—keeping a good distance, however, from the bed.

The Authorities Plan against Other Infections

The frustrating effect of continuous epidemics on industry and agriculture roused the anger of influential people. From the fourteenth century onwards, the authorities launched determined attacks on all fronts against plague and other infections.

Official recognition was given to the importance of cleanliness. In the reign of Edward the First, the first Sanitary Act was passed, forbidding the pollution of rivers, ditches and open spaces; this signified that the people could no longer dump their refuse anywhere, and in some cities rubbish collections were organised, and the people levied for the cost of the work. The authorities also undertook to empty and clean ponds and small dams at regular times, and arranged public places where housewives could bring the family wash.

The enthusiasm for cleanliness grew. Every citizen was expected to clean the pavement outside his house on each saint's day, and charity and public bath-houses were set up to encourage personal hygiene. In the monasteries and large houses the luxury of a private bath-tub was introduced, and Saturday night gradually became accepted as bath-night, and workers and apprentices were released from their jobs an hour earlier for this good cause.

Throughout Europe the struggle for public health was taken up; Italian and German citizens laid the foundations of a sanitary law which made sure that at least the water supply was clean and the streets free from objectionable accumulations of dirt; Vienna and Milan set up health councils with power to see that the sanitary laws were respected.

Undoubtedly some improvements were gained, but it was not a one-sided battle. The growth of industry and towns was quicker than the slow machinery of the law, and sometimes the open space reserved for the dumping of refuse would become almost overnight the site of new hutments for the expanding population. The general state of public health is sensitively recorded by the average expectation of life at any period; the famous nineteenth-century social reformer, Sir Edwin Chadwick, estimated that children born in the year 1550 could expect to survive on an average until they were eight and a half years old; in Geneva, a medieval town with a worse record of overcrowding than most, so many babies died at birth that the average expectation of life was only four years and nine months. From that estimate alone one can draw a fair picture of the many battles that medical science and civic co-operation were compelled to wage for the sake of human happiness and well-being.

Nevertheless, the worst of the afflictions that had almost overwhelmed mankind in the first 1,000 years of the new European civilisation were under control by about the fourteenth century. Men no longer suffered so frequently from diseases following on prolonged famine; agriculture and land-drainage had been so improved that minimum needs at least could be supplied. An island like Britain had developed sufficient overseas trade to be able to import the foodstuffs it lacked. A bare existence was still the lot of the poor workers, but a social protection, however flimsy, had at least been erected for the sick and infirm. Living together in a complex society, people had come to understand that it was in the general interest to provide some form of welfare for those who failed to support themselves. To some people, it was a moral obligation to give charity, to others an unwelcome levy enforced by the authorities; but society as a whole had learnt that if too many of the members of the community are allowed to go under, the whole structure could be dragged down; and so organisations were created which later gave rise to the Poor Laws, the Public Health services, and the Health Insurance system of modern times.

The "Unclean" Disease

Next to the "Black Death" the history of the Middle Ages is haunted by the figure of the outcast leper, ringing his warning bell and crying out his own death sentence, "Unclean, unclean".

The outward signs of the disease were familiar enough to the medieval citizens; the thickened skin, the hoarse voice, the many foul-smelling sores that spread and finally rotted the miserable victim, were enough in themselves to keep healthy people at a distance; yet in spite of the almost hysterical terror which the disease provoked in people, it spread at a furious rate over Europe and England.

There was a common view that such an affliction must be the result of sinful behaviour, and the moral attitude of the Church towards this "unclean" disease added authority to the medical view that isolation was the only way to prevent its spread. Medical opinion held that leprosy was inherited, and could be spread by contact, and doctors gave no hope of recovery. It was thought sufferers had probably provoked their condition by dirty habits and sexual licence, or even by eating poisonous food or not enough fresh vegetables and fruit.

Medical treatment, therefore, was simply designed to exclude the condemned person as effectively as possible from everyday life. Like a criminal, he lost all his civic rights, was forbidden to marry and could be divorced. He could not speak to anyone or use public fountains or inns; when he ventured into the market places, he had to keep sounding the warning rattle, and dared only point with a rod at anything he wished to buy. As a concession to the spiritual welfare of the leper, small windows were built into the walls of churches, so that the outcast could see, if not share, the religious ceremony.

Lepers were considered to be under the protection of three Saints, Francis, Elizabeth and Louis, but the Church finally provided a more practical protection with the charitable bequests and taxes levied for the purpose, by building special leper houses and colonies so that people could be kept off the roads and prevented from unwittingly spreading the disease so universally feared. At one time there were as many as 20,000 such leper-houses on the Continent, and over 200 in England; and this undoubtedly helped to check the spread of the disease and keep it under some control.

There was one law for the rich and one for the poor even in these institutions. Most wealthy citizens who had the disease were allowed to remain in their own homes, but if they went into the leper-houses, they could bring with them all their usual comforts, soft bedding, good clothing and silver tableware. Those who could not pay for such luxuries received only the harsh treatment reserved for the poor.

It is clear this disease reached its peak during the periods of social upheaval following the Continental wars. Voltaire, the French philosopher, commented cynically on these medieval wars: "Of all that we gained by the Crusades and of all that we have taken, leprosy was the only thing we kept."

The Doctors Tackle Disease

Medieval communities and their medical advisers were kept fully occupied in the field of public health, battling with what must have seemed an endless series of epidemics.

These afflictions, like the famine pestilences of the early part of the Middle Ages, could produce an effect as demoralising to the whole population as modern warfare can today. After a famine, typhus or influenza would rage, leaving behind whole areas devastated, with homes empty and silent and inhabitants dead, or their bodies rotting in the unharvested fields. The survivors, who were often outnumbered by the dead, took ravenously what food they could, horses, dogs, and even, as shown by irrefutable evidence, other human beings, especially defenceless children.

What could the doctors do? Their ignorance of the causes of disease was paralleled by the bigoted attitude of those in authority towards rational scientific enquiry. Yet there was no escaping the reality of the epidemics and their effects, and some very practical advances were made in communal action to isolate infection and stop it from spreading.

An almost complete state of emergency existed, and the leisurely pursuit of the study of general ill health slowed down to a crawling pace. Western Church dogma also had an inhibiting effect on new thought, and in these circumstances, contemporary medical knowledge made relatively rapid advances in the rising empire of Arabia. From the seventh to the twelfth century Arabia increased in power and importance, and with the usual acquisitiveness of new empires, it collected not only the wealth, but much of the learning of its neighbours.

Despite the destructiveness of successive wars and conquests, much of the best of Greek classical thought was still preserved in manuscripts and in the remains of the once great library at Alexandria. Syrian translations provided the link between Greece and Arabia, and a valuable contribution was made in this part of the world by Jewish physicians gathering medical knowledge from all the lands where they were exiled and showing themselves to be especially expert at diagnosis.

Arabian Doctors take the Lead

The Arabs were particularly shrewd and observant, and continued the progressive tradition of Greece and Rome, although magic ritual still clung to the practice and beliefs of the mass of the people.

Arabian physicians adopted the methods of Hippocrates and Galen, and gave clearly detailed descriptions of many common diseases such as pleurisy, diabetes, worm infection and venereal diseases. The description of pleurisy reads like a Greek or even a modern case history:

"The patient has a continuous fever, and a sharp pain between the ribs, sometimes felt only when he breathes strongly; his breathing is rapid and difficult, his pulse weak and rapid, and his cough, at first dry, may later be accompanied by sputum, when it signifies that the lung also is affected."

The Arabian physicians made an important distinction between smallpox and measles, and were not misled by the fact that the rash may appear the same in both diseases: they pointed out that excitement, anxiety and nausea were more frequent in measles, while the pain in the back was more common in smallpox. The more serious disease of smallpox was kept isolated in hospitals or pest-houses.

The Greeks had established the traditional use of a large number of tried and tested herbal remedies and drugs, and the Arabian pharmacists were able to add to these from the natural abundance of the gardens of the East. The perfumes and spices of the Orient were skilfully blended to serve the healing art: amber, musk, manna, cloves, nutmeg, tamarind, camphor, senna, cassia, Chinese ginger, betel-nut, sandalwood; over 1,400 were classified and studied, and so provided a further basis for a science of chemistry. New remedies were introduced, such as animal gut for ligatures and mercurial ointments, which are still employed today. General treatment followed the old simple methods of enemas, purges and bleedings; the cautery was often used with too much enthusiasm and must frequently have done more harm than good.

Arabian medicine included advanced surgery, but this was left to the lower medical grades, for the old tradition still held that it was an unworthy occupation. The Mohammedan religion shared with the Christian a horror of the dissections of the human body, and consequently little progress was made in the study of anatomy. Despite this drawback, all the well-known operations were carried out, including those for hernia, haemorrhoids and goitre, and cancer of the breast and the womb. The Arabian doctors showed skill and originality which provided a stimulus to further medical advances.

In internal operations, they held the edges of the wound together by using large ants whose natural reaction was to fix their legs powerfully into the flesh; and then the surgeon cut off their heads, retaining the joining effect for the medical purpose of forming a strong bridge. Plastic surgery was a skilled art with the Arabs, who effectively remedied defects of the skin, eyelids, forehead, nose and cheeks. They introduced the use of silver instead of bronze for some instruments, and their dental treatment included the provision of false teeth made of beef bone.

The patient was given a simple but effective anaesthetic. Sponges were soaked in a narcotic such as opium or mandragora; they were then dried, and when the patient was prepared for operation they were placed in very hot water, and he breathed in relief from pain with the rising vapour.

The Arabians organised a very efficient hospital service for their times. Hospitals were built in the most suitable locality; according to a legend the choice of a site was made by one physician in a unique way. He hung up pieces of meat in various parts of the city, and finally decided on the locality where the meat had stayed fresh for the longest time, indicating that in that part of the city there was the least danger of contamination from the mysterious source which caused putrefaction and disease.

By the tenth century A.D., every Moslem city had its own hospital. An important town like Baghdad had sixty hospitals with out-patients' departments which distributed medicines. The hospitals were spacious, with wards for different ailments, and fountains pleasantly refreshing the atmosphere. Male and female nurses looked after the patients under the supervision of eminent physicians.

A very important factor of this well-organised hospital service was the absence of any charge for treatment, but so far removed was it from the cold charity of other lands that minstrels and dancers were employed to cheer patients during their convalescence; and on being discharged each patient was given five pieces of gold so that he could fully recover before returning to work.

This was largely the work of a progressively-minded physician of the Arabian empire who was given the task of organising the entire service, and was fortunate to receive generous official backing from the Caliph of the time. A serious effort was also made to establish a permanent foundation for training future doctors and physicians. Laboratories and apothecaries' shops were established, and courses of study organised with examinations in chemistry, pharmacy, optics and mathematics.

The finest achievements of Arabic medicine of the tenth century were crystallised in the work and personality of Avicenna, a native of Bukhara, and a doctor whose wisdom and skill place him among the immortal names in medicine. His great work, the *Canon*, was a vast encyclopaedia of medical knowledge which served as a text-book in many countries for several hundred years. His advice extended beyond the mere treatment of a sick patient, and he was concerned with the effects on health of the environment, climate, water supply and emotional background of the individual. Avicenna's approach to medicine was positive and confident, a quality which has a lasting significance, in spite of the limitations of his times.

Nevertheless, the prevailing mood of the Middle Ages was closer to a belief in witchcraft than to reason. Arabian physicians, like their colleagues all over Europe, were as much conjurers and magicians as doctors. They were reflecting the general trend in which rational and irrational elements struggled for expression, sometimes in conflict, sometimes side by side, without apparent contradiction in the eyes of the people. For example, in the very hospital where the patient was receiving the most modern scientific treatment for his complaint, fifty holy speakers were employed to keep up a continuous recital night and day, repeating prayers from the Koran in order to hasten the cure.

Medieval Medicine and Mysticism

Medieval doctors in all lands compensated for their lack of real knowledge by an opulent outward appearance, which, although it often angered more intelligent observers, suitably impressed the ignorant. In the East the worth of a physician was measured by the height of his turban and the length of his sleeves. He often had a number of tricks hidden up them, including charms and "magic" inks with which he wrote his prescriptions. He was also cunning enough to hire a few spies who gave him information about the patients, who were duly impressed by the doctor's "insight". The Italian doctor strutted about in rich robes trimmed with jewels and ermine, his external worth out of all proportion to his inner value.

Such doctors had confused ideas about the functions of the body and its organs. Typical of their fanciful theories was the statement that the heart was the prince of the body, the lungs the fan of the heart, and the liver the seat of the soul; medical remedies were presented in a similar fictional form. Pills and potions were to be taken "when Jupiter and Venus were in the ascendant". Cupping was best performed when the moon was on the wane, preferably "on the seventeenth of the moon, and on a Tuesday".

From primitive times, an almost magical significance has been attached to the excretions of the body. In general the medieval physician drew his conclusions from studying the blood, sputum and urine, paying attention to the colour, odour and density, but there was little rational understanding in his mind. From the layers of sediment in a specimen of urine he concluded that murkiness of the top layer indicated disease of the head, and of the lower layer, disease of the genital organs. Exploiting popular credulity to the full, these doctors claimed they could diagnose everything, including pregnancy, from an examination of the urine. Many a true word is spoken in jest, and today urine can be tested to prove pregnancy, but there the resemblance ends.

There was a continuous confusion between rational and mystical methods. Bleeding was a common treatment, but it was determined by astrological considerations, such as the right day and season, as well as the patient's age and temperament. Medieval treatises devote pages to lengthy discussions on such irrelevancies.

The physicians, necromancers and apothecaries of the Middle Ages were obsessed with two ambitions: to discover a formula that would turn all base metal to gold, and to create an "elixir of life" that would cure all ailments and make man for ever young. Engrossed in such futile aims they ignored the real problems of everyday life.

A New Hope in Europe

The Arabian school of medicine, for all its oriental exuberance, did not profoundly influence the trend of medieval thought, but it did keep alive the old classical scientific manuscripts, which were copied and re-copied by industrious monks throughout Europe. The monastery at Monte Cassino (which, having risen above the early barbarism of European history, was shattered in the new barbarism of 1939-45), served as a centre for spreading knowledge throughout the Middle Ages.

The ecclesiastical atmosphere placed a restraint on the medical outlook of these writers and teachers, but in the twelfth and thirteenth centuries, the dim light of scientific enquiry suddenly brightened in an obscure corner of Italy, where there was an old-established medical school at the little seaside town of Salerno, near Naples.

Although they followed the mistaken theories of Galen, studied anatomy solely from examinations of pigs, and based their diagnosis only on a study of the pulse and urine, the good common sense which had characterised the Hippocratic physicians came to the surface once more. These doctors, like the Greeks, seemed suddenly to come out of doors into fresh air, after long midnight sessions of the magico-mystical ritual in which all other medieval physicians were steeped. They began to study diseases at first hand as Hippocrates had taught, and practised simple therapeutic treatment based on sensible rules of health, in place of the usual mumbo-jumbo.

The teachings of this school were embodied in a long poem, the *Regimen sanitatis Salernitanum*, which established itself as the practical handbook of all the medieval physicians in Europe, up to the time of the Renaissance. Its precise and simple advice must have proved a refreshing source of information after the muddled outpourings of medieval sorcery.

The poem counsels moderation in all things, and an even and natural way of life. Practical rules of health are given:

> *Rise early in the morn, and straight remember*
> *With water cold to wash your hands and eyes,*
> *In gentle fashion reaching every member,*
> *And to refresh your brain when you arise* ...

The healthy man cleans his teeth, goes for walks and keeps out of draughts, and avoids living near bad smells. Wine, women and baths bring health and happiness if taken in moderation.

Medical methods are dealt with (the pithy Latin being translated in the seventeenth century into English verse).

To the surgeon:

> *Make your incision large and not too deep*
> *That blood have speedy issue with the fume*
> *So that from the sinews you all hurt do keep* ...

The poem describes the effects of the common foods and drinks, and gives advice on bleeding and suitable remedies, mainly herbal, for headache, toothache and indigestion.

Medical thought benefited greatly from the wide diffusion of this re-birth of the Greek idea, but it was clearly advice which could be taken seriously only by people who were in a position to choose where they lived, what they ate, and how they enjoyed their hours of leisure.

The school of Salerno was the beginning. Other centres of learning were founded, expressing the renewal of man's interest in finding sensible answers to the problems of an increasingly complex way of life. In Montpellier and Bologna, Paris and Padua, the young men crowded the newly established universities to learn the sum of knowledge on all subjects; anatomy, physiology and surgery sharing pride of place with law, theology and philosophy. From A.D. 1200 to the end of the Middle Ages the foundation stones were laid of over eighty European universities.

Most of these universities were presided over by highly placed clerics, and the licence to teach was given in the name of the Pope or well-established Church authority. The students paid for their tuition, and lived in the colleges with their tutors who were divided between the lay and clerical professions.

With the growth of medical schools and much-needed hospitals a new outlook was provided for medical teaching and knowledge, based less on surmise than on the regular study of clinical cases. The importance of anatomical study was recognised, and European universities such as those at Padua, Venice and Florence dissected bodies of executed criminals handed over by the authorities for this purpose. This break with tradition was essential for the progress of surgery. As an eminent surgeon of the fourteenth century wrote: "It is necessary that the surgeon especially know anatomy, because without anatomy one can do nothing in surgery." This may seem self-evident to modern minds, but much prejudice had to be broken down before human dissection became a common part of training in surgery.

Medieval Medicine—the Hard Way Forward

Man, in his struggle to live and to keep healthy, had been cast down into confusion after the fall of the slave empires. At the beginning of medieval times, he had clung desperately to Roman medicine, with all its fallacies about "humours", and the mystical qualities of blood and urine, as indoctrinated by Galen, the greatest Roman physician of them all.

Medieval man had advanced very little beyond the Greeks and the Romans, with his amulets, incantations, "cuppings", and bleedings; nevertheless, the tremendous struggle waged by the whole community against the evils of famine and epidemics had led them onward through error and confusion to a better understanding of hygiene and precautionary methods for good health.

The skill of man's hands had expressed itself best in simple surgical operations, which limited knowledge had permitted surgeons to undertake. Arabian surgeons had mastered the delicate operation of puncturing and needling the lens for cataract; the dim-sighted were fitted with spectacles; and in general man had learnt that with more knowledge he could battle more effectively with disease.

However, his methods were still a weird blend of witchcraft and practical skill. Mysterious coloured liquids in the pharmacists' shops might be useful potions based on herbal recipes, or some utterly disgusting concoction such as bile of vipers or spermatic fluid of frogs: it was all one to the medieval patient; perhaps he had even greater confidence in the more unpleasant prescriptions, in the belief derived from primitive times that cures come from opposites.

But, as in all periods, only the basically sound ideas could stand the test of practice: and towards the end of the Middle Ages, medicine and mankind were emerging from the darkness into which they had plunged in the early social upheavals of their times; there were tremendous changes ahead—and tremendous problems; which at last they were preparing to face.

Chapter Six

THE RENAISSANCE

Science and Medicine Reawaken

THE Old World had made contact with the New. At the opening of the period later honoured by the name of the Renaissance, America had been discovered, and the Cape of Good Hope was rounded, bringing vast new colonies within European domination. The half-forgotten trade routes to East India and China were re-opened, and the rising class of merchants in Europe saw before them an alluring prospect of markets. To satisfy the needs of these markets, it was necessary to improve manufacture and transport by land and sea. The influential burghers of the Middle Ages emerged as the rising merchant class, and they concentrated in their hands the new industries which were replacing the craft guilds with their small output.

The extension of world markets coincided with an energetic development of communications and manufacture. This added to the possessions of the merchants, and by the close of the Renaissance, all classes in society had surrendered to the supremacy of the new capitalist class. The rural areas conceded leadership to the towns, and the undeveloped nations of the world were subjected to the more advanced ones.

This great change first became most marked in England in the fourteenth century. The demand for increased output of goods was already undermining the complete dependence of the serf on the manor; the rising demand of the Flemish market for English wool had a profound effect on the system of serfdom. Within a short time the serf was giving a far poorer return for his keep than a well-fleeced sheep. Soon the people were driven off the land in thousands, by the inhuman laws of the Enclosures; and flocks of sheep fattened on the rich English soil, almost entirely given over to pasture.

The renewed interest in science, philosophy and medicine which marked the Renaissance was most successful in the most economically advanced country, and England is therefore predominant in any discussion of medical and scientific achievements from the sixteenth and seventeenth centuries onwards.

The expansion of commerce and industry which broke completely through the feudal restraints also undermined scholastic and religious dogmas. There was a growing urgency to know more about science, chemistry, and the natural laws of the universe. The new problems presented by the growing industries and ever-extending communications had to be solved by a rational and practical approach; mystical speculation could no longer masquerade as science. The philosophical dogmatism which had ruled for centuries lost ground in the developing universities, where the new outlook was of intense scientific curiosity closely linked to real experience. There was a revived interest in the teachings of Ancient Greece and Rome which evoked a sympathetic response in this new scientific era.

The re-birth of learning was not, however, painless. In the sixteenth century, Copernicus, the Polish astronomer, was the first to realise that the earth was not the centre of the universe, but he hesitated for many years before he dared to make public his knowledge. His book *On the Revolution of the Celestial Spheres* was published in 1543, the year he died, many years after he had first recorded his revolutionary theory. Copernicus died in bed, but the judgment of the Church, which he had feared, fell upon one of his followers, Giordano Bruno, who chose to be burnt at the stake rather than deny what he knew to be a scientific fact.

But the practical needs of the time could not be ignored. Navigation required a more exact astronomy; machines could be enlarged and improved only with the help of physics and mathematics; and industrial processes faced difficulties which stimulated the science of chemistry to new adventures.

In the seventeenth century, Galileo invented a wonderful new instrument, the telescope, which opened his eyes to new horizons. Despite the animosity and persecution of the Church, he pursued his study of the laws which govern the universe. He expressed his attitude neatly when he stated: "Nature is written in mathematical symbols."

At the same time, Sir Francis Bacon continued the rational, scientific approach by underlining the need to note carefully facts connected with experiment, and to draw conclusions from the results of experience and not from speculative theories only. He stated that his aim was "to extend more widely the limits of the power and the greatness of man". Recorded facts, new observations and experimental results were to be collected and tabulated so that the connection between phenomena and the general laws of nature would become apparent.

The sciences of astronomy and mathematics were extended still further by the work of Johannes Kepler, who discovered the laws of movements of planets, and by the renowned Sir Isaac Newton, whose discovery of the law of gravity and findings in mechanics and mathematics brought rational science to a point where mere guesswork based on superstitions could no longer be accepted blindly. Aristotle and Galen were finally placed on the marble pedestal of antiquity, and the religious universe was consigned to myth and legend.

The new learning was exchanged between thinking people of every land, by a development which was as important to the Renaissance as the discovery of writing had been to the Ancient Egyptians. In England printing was introduced by William Caxton at the end of the fifteenth century, and from that time new ideas and formulas could be conveyed to hundreds of thousands of people, renewed and enriched with the thoughts of many men, as speedily as books could be run off the press.

In such an encouraging atmosphere the arts, too, began to relax and move beyond the formal stiffness of the medieval era. Literature, sculpture and painting took on new forms, more alive, closer to people and reality. With the sciences making such progress, medicine, following the same rational path, also began to move away decisively from the dim half-world of magic to the reality of practical experiment. Anatomists, physicians and surgeons learned from physicists, mathematicians and chemists, and in their turn were able to contribute to the general fund and to the science of sciences, philosophy.

The Human Body

Of all the mysteries that had intrigued man since early days, his own body had been the greatest puzzle and had proved the most difficult to decipher. Fear, superstition and religion had inhibited

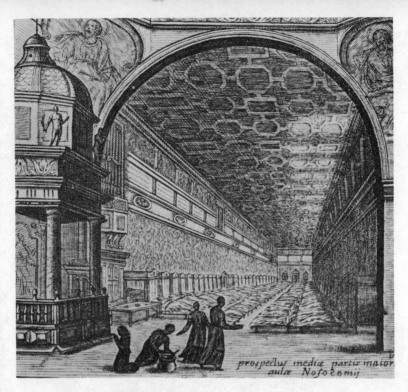

Hospital ward, San Spirito, Rome (seventeenth century).

Mr Howard offering relief to prisoners, 1787.

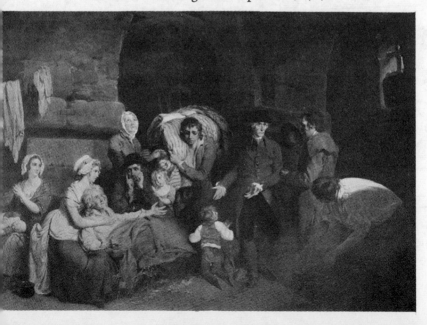

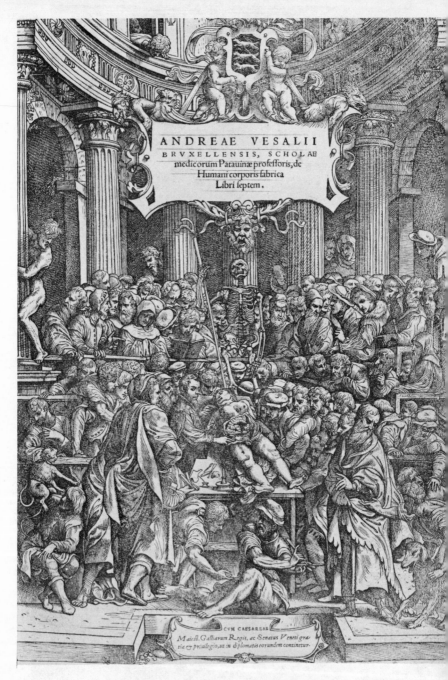

Title page to Vesalius' *De Humani Corporis Fabrica*.

serious study of the workings of the body, but with the birth of the
new commercial age, scientific enquiry was stimulated, and very
soon attention was directed with fresh curiosity to the study of man
himself.

In the fifteenth century, Leonardo da Vinci trained himself to become a painter and sculptor by studying human anatomy in detail.
Without this knowledge, he said, "artists would make their nudes
wooden and without grace". The whole scope of medicine gained
by the better understanding of anatomy and physiology which followed his pioneering work in dissection. Leonardo's notebooks are
not only works of art, but also works which were of great scientific
value in their time, particularly in his exact drawings of bones, muscles,
joints, tendons, the heart, the lungs, and other parts of the body.
Many false beliefs about the human body and its functions were ended
by the work of this great man of the Renaissance, who approached
the problems of his art in the best scientific tradition and brought to
scientific enquiry the imagination and foresight of a great artist.

Once the prohibitions on dissecting the human body had been
ignored, further advances in anatomy could be made. Vesalius dominated the lecture room of the University at Padua in the sixteenth
century, and his personality and teaching spread through Europe.
His carefully planned work on the human body was directed against
the dogmatic errors of the classical Roman, Galen, whose teachings
had ruled medical thought for many generations.

The circulation of the blood was one of the principle medical
enigmas that had not been satisfactorily answered. Galen had created
confusion by maintaining that the blood must inevitably pass from
the right to the left chamber of the heart through "invisible" pores.
Vesalius confidently made public the denial that many doctors must
have privately considered. He said, "I do not see how even the
smallest amount of blood could pass from the right ventricle to the
left through the septum". All who had handled the septum could see
that it was an impenetrable wall between the two sides of the heart.
Vesalius based his opinions on an extensive dissection of dogs, mice
and other small animals, as well as on more spectacular work on
human bodies.

The year 1543 was a notable one for the publishing world, and more so for the world of science. First there was Copernicus, writing *On the Revolutions of the Celestial Spheres*, and then Vesalius, with his masterpiece *On the Workings of the Human Body*. The book had illustrations taken from copperplate engravings by Calcar, a gifted pupil of Titian (it is also likely that some were executed by Titian); the body was depicted in motion as it is in life, and the book still lives today as a valuable work on anatomy. Understandably, Vesalius, although well ahead of many of his time, made a number of anatomical mistakes, particularly as he had no rational concept of the circulation of the blood. However, he blazed the way for the many skilled anatomists who followed him.

The Advance of Surgery

Some advances had been made in surgical technique on the many battlefields of the Roman Empire, and with the discovery of gunpowder new varieties of wounds were often the reward of the crusaders of the "holy" wars of the sixteenth and seventeenth centuries.

Ambroise Paré, a surgeon who was able and willing to learn from the advances in anatomy, demonstrated that surgery could be raised to a more respected place in medicine. Surgery had for long been classed as a trade, with a status between that of the barber and the butcher; and often it was the barber who wielded the surgical razor.

Like many others, Paré practised on the battlefield, and he had an unusual experience which proved of value to all who suffered from wounds. The Arabs taught that bleeding could be stopped only by pouring boiling oil on to the wound, and so this had been practised for centuries. After one battle, Paré found to his dismay that there was not enough oil for all the infected wounds, so some soldiers had to rest content with an improvised dressing of a mixture of eggs, oil of roses, and turpentine. Paré spent a sleepless night, expecting to find these patients dead in the morning, but to his relief and astonishment those who had not had the supposed advantage of the boiling oil treatment were less feverish and in a much better condition than those who had had it. He resolved "never more to burn cruelly poor men with gunshot wounds". Seeking further relief for his patients, he learned to tie arteries at the point where they were torn and bleeding, thus avoiding the use of the cautery.

The ancient doctrine "that diseases not curable by iron are curable by fire" had been followed blindly and religiously for hundreds of years. Paré proved by practical experience that this was false. He fought against the medical practices based on old dogmas, such as applying plasters with unpleasant ingredients, including ground-up frogs, worms and vipers to wounds presumed poisoned, on the basis that one poison counteracted another.

Paré had a positive approach to his patients; he spent much time and ingenuity in devising artificial limbs, and he was always moved by deep humanity and a proper sense of values. Once when he was congratulated on the successful outcome of a difficult case, he made a reply that was long remembered, containing good counsel for the over-confident: "I treated him, God cured him."

The New Medicine

The current critical and rebellious mood expressed itself with force through the person of "Bombastus" Paracelsus von Hohenheim. He came from Germany to study at the Italian universities, but he soon antagonised everyone by his refusal to follow unquestioningly the traditional medicine. Like Hippocrates, he insisted that experience was the best teacher, and he strongly influenced practising physicians all over Europe to adopt the clinical "bedside" approach, to the great benefit of the patient. He parted from his Italian colleagues with some anger on both sides, and as a lecturer he insisted on teaching in the language of the country, leaving Latin to the greybeards who clothed ancient thoughts in an ancient tongue. He is reported to have commenced a lecture by publicly burning text-books of Galen and others. Paracelsus was too outspoken and too critical to be popular, and he cynically commented, "I pleased no one, except the sick whom I healed".

Paracelsus was in all ways a man of his times. He expressed the spirit of the Renaissance through his uncompromising attitude towards the old theoreticians whose views were being discredited by rational investigation. But just as the Middle Ages threw long shadows which the light of the Renaissance did not completely remove, so Paracelsus, despite his modern approach, reflected in his theories the old magic of the astrologers and alchemists. So strong in criticising others, he thought that he was above criticism, being moved by the Holy Spirit which illuminated his thoughts; and he became more deeply involved in mysticism. He believed that living matter and all metals share common components, salt, sulphur and mercury, and that the colour of a drug had some relation to the type of disease for which it could best be used. For example, he taught that gold was of use in cardiac diseases because yellow was the colour also of the sun, which rules the heart. This compound of alchemy and imagination induced Paracelsus to recommend spotted skins of lizards for malignant tumours, decoctions of blood-red poppies for wounded soldiers, and walnut shells for head injuries because of the resemblance of the kernel to the contour of the brain. He treated plague with medicine made from frogs because both were equally disgusting and before an epidemic twenty frogs sat one on the other, representing a symbolic warning of the depth of human bodies to be flung to a heap in mass graves.

Yet Paracelsus will be remembered, for in spite of his errors he actively led the forward march of medicine.

Not "Why" but "How"

A most important change had taken place when medical investigators began to put to the test how different organs of the body worked. Medieval philosophers had wandered down roads of fantasy leading nowhere. The new experiments soon produced impressive results which encouraged new forms of inquiry.

The great puzzle, how the blood flowed through the body, was a little less obscure; the circulation of blood through the lungs had been traced, and how blood reached and left the heart through the great vessels; but the essence of the classical theory that the liver was the centre of the circulation was still accepted, until the appearance in the seventeenth century of one of the greatest scientists of all, the Englishman, William Harvey.

Harvey went to Italy to study, and when he returned to medical practice in England, he continued his experiments with meticulous care. He soon came to the momentous conclusion that the blood moves continuously, and always in one direction, a solution to many problems which had baffled medical men for thousands of years;

Harvey did not publish the results of his scientific inquiry for a further thirteen years, but when he did so, he had established irrefutably that the blood circulated from a central organ, the heart.

He was ignorant of the presence of capillaries linking the arteries and the veins, but he deduced there was some form of union. However, he was still undecided on whether the task of circulation was the nourishing or the cooling of the body.

Harvey had pushed experiment as far as it could go, with no equipment other than the naked eye. But just as the telescope revealed distant stars to the discerning observation of Galileo, so the microscope opened up a new universe of tiny living matter to Malpighi, who, four years after Harvey's death, solved the mystery of the union of the blood vessels. He placed the simple and transparent tissue of the lung of a frog under the microscope, and at last the connecting link of the capillaries joining arteries and veins was visible, completing the picture of the circulation of the blood so brilliantly described by William Harvey.

The microscope fascinated, as it still does, people with inquisitive minds; it was held with a passionate fervour in the imagination of a Dutch merchant, Leeuwenhoek, who for nearly sixty years continued to grind his own lenses with ever greater skill, so that he could see in his insatiable curiosity many things hidden from the ordinary view.

What had begun as a hobby became an absorbing passion, as through his lens he was stimulated by glimpses of living organisms never before seen by any man.

Leeuwenhoek described the blood cells of man and animals and the thinnest walls of the smallest blood vessels, so making the study of the circulation even more precise. Everything be brought under his lens revealed a world within a world; he perceived the composition of living tissue, the structure of protozoa and spermatozoa. Then one day he smeared some of the film from his teeth on to a slide, and as a result described "little animals more numerous than the population in the Netherlands, and moving about in a most delightful manner".

Bacteria, after thousands of years of invisibility, were at last revealed by the microscope as man's closest living companions; but whether friend or enemy was not even considered yet. That came at a much later stage, when Pasteur performed his famous experiments.

New Theories for Old

Scientists no longer considered man to be a divine mystery, any more than they did the universe. Physicists and astronomers demonstrated that they could weigh and measure the earth with mathematical precision. Chemical laboratories had not yet cleared their shelves of the alchemists' coloured liquids and magic mixtures, so medical research adapted to its own uses the mathematical principles which had brought so much progress in other sciences.

Sixteenth and seventeenth-century investigators into the structure of man thought of him as a machine and carried out experiments on this basis. Typical was the work of one, Sanctorius, who made a special balance in which he ate and slept, carefully noting the effect of his actions on his weight; he made an important observation on the continuous though unnoticed loss of moisture through the skin. He suggested that all should possess such a simple machine so that they could guard against irregularities in the intake of food, which he considered the cause of most diseases. Sanctorius invented a thermometer for taking the heat of the body, which was an unwieldy forerunner of the now familiar instrument.

One professor of mathematics explained man in terms of mechanics. He correctly illustrated how muscles move limbs as strings and levers move mechanical objects, and he saw all the functions of the body as working in similar ways. What made the machine work? His answer was: something intangible—the soul; for when it leaves the body, all movement ceases.

Another scientist, Baglivi, carried this theory even further, and described activities of the body by comparison with the many machines: the teeth, as scissors; the stomach, a grinding mill; the heart and blood-vessels, a water-works system; and the chest-wall, bellows. Despite this fanciful speculation, his practical work as a doctor was more realistic; and he did excellent work as a clinician. His advice to students was in direct line with all rational physicians since Hippocrates: "Let the young know that they will never find a more interesting, more instructive book than the patient himself."

At this stage, philosophy took up the challenge to construct a comprehensive and unifying account of the knowledge of man and the universe. As all the scientific studies had been along the lines of how things moved and worked, it was logical that philosophy should repeat this mechanical approach. Descartes spoke for his age when he described man as a machine. He regarded all activities as physical motions which could be examined precisely, and he understood correctly that the brain was the controlling organ. But how does man know himself? How is he aware of the outside world? This was beyond the scope of the "man the machine" explanation, so philosophy went into the opposite camp to find an answer. Descartes, the mechanist, said: "I think, therefore I am." His mechanical world had to be created and set in motion, so he was forced to go outside his own theory and accept the idea of a Divine Spirit which showed itself through living matter. He did not, however, concede to animals the personal soul which he bestowed on man.

Since the current philosophy maintained that man, in so far as he could be studied, was to be conceived as a machine, medical theory was directed towards explaining everything about the body in terms of mathematics and mechanics; the slower evolution of chemistry and biology had not yet illuminated the chemical and organic processes.

The experimenters began to weigh and measure the various parts of man as if he were so much brick, cement and lead piping. So it was reckoned that the muscles moving the thumb weighed 122 grains and they were estimated to develop a power of 3,270 pounds; accordingly the stomach, although weighing only eight ounces, could generate a force of 117,088 pounds, increasing to 461,219 pounds when the muscles of the abdomen and diaphragm were working full strength. Fruitless efforts were made to calculate the weight of an individual spermatozoon. The most logical absurdity, however, that arose from the school of "physical" medicine, was the mathematical theory which worked out the span of life depending on the number of times a man's heart had been geared to beat. So that if a person had a heart fixed to last seventy years provided it beat at an average rate of sixty times a minute, then too much excitement which raised the heart beats to an average of seventy-five a minute would automatically determine the man's end at fifty-six years.

Amidst all these exciting and modern experiments, chemistry could not remain for long immersed in the centuries' old traditions based on the alchemist's four principal elements, earth, fire, air and water. The English chemist, Robert Boyle, laid the foundation of the science of chemistry. In company with a number of other scientific men, he formed "The Invisible College" (which later became the Royal Society), whose purpose was to conduct experiments and draw conclusions only from what they had learned by practice. Boyle was in the forefront of many important experiments; he established that air has substance and weight by placing a cat in a vessel and then causing it to show signs of suffocation by removing the air with a pump (so proving that breathing did not depend on some mysterious spirit).

This new movement in chemistry was taken up eagerly, as it proved an alternative explanation to mechanical formulas. The old theory of the four humours of the body took on a more up-to-date interpretation, with bodily changes related to the saliva, the pancreatic juice and the bile. One professor of medicine took this to the extreme of suggesting that diseases could be analysed and treated chemically with such absurd logic as, "If all the blood is black, that indicates that acid predominates; while if it is red, the bile predominates. In the former case it is necessary to diminish the acid in the body and the blood; in the latter to diminish the bile and weaken its strength." The enthusiasts of this school of thought explained man's state of health entirely in terms of chemical changes, and they compared the role of the physician to that of the brewer controlling the process of fermentation in the vat, preventing or correcting any irregularities.

The philosophic pendulum which had swung so violently in the mechanistic direction swung back to the opposite extreme. To some philosophers, known as "Vitalists", the law which controlled man and the universe was the law of "the sensitive soul", a vital spirit which worked through the passive machine, the body. Illness and disease simply expressed through the body a disorder of the spirit or soul.

The Renaissance in Medical Study

The way forward for medicine was clearly the way of investigation and experiment, and the physicians once and for all turned their backs on the old dogma. There was not yet a solid basis of the science of medicine, but there was an important advance in the methods of careful clinical observation, as taught in particular by Thomas Sydenham, who, in the seventeenth century, was considered "the English Hippocrates".

Sydenham proposed a significant departure from the old method of treating the sick on the basis that the balance of "humours" had been disturbed, ignoring the specific disease which was the real cause of the trouble. He returned to the older concept of disease as an entity which had invaded the body, and he developed the principle that treatment should help the body to get rid of the unhealthy substances through the blood.

In the past, a few diseases had been recognised in the general confusion of symptoms. Rhazes of Arabia had distinguished measles from smallpox, and leprosy had been accepted since Biblical times as a clearly-defined illness. It was Sydenham who first made a systematic study of symptoms, and assigned them to specific illnesses and disorders, and so by obtaining a better understanding of the case, made treatment more simple and effective. He clearly distinguished between scarlet fever, measles and smallpox, but he encountered difficulties when he refused to accept any guiding medical theory. He had noted 1,800 different symptoms, and like Hippocrates, was forced in spite of his intentions to fall back on old theories to save him from the impossibility of treating so many different diseases. The Great Plague of London in 1665 gave him wide experience and much cause for thought, and he finally came back to the theory of "epidemic constitutions", namely, the idea of atmospheric or cosmic influences working on contagious diseases in all sorts of unpredictable ways; and he surmised that some infectious diseases might be spread from miasmas out of the bowels of the earth.

From the seventeenth century onwards, the advance of knowledge continues almost unbroken, from one country to another, from one advanced-thinking physician to another, each gaining from the progress won by other workers in medical research. This does not mean, of course, that the most advanced knowledge was automatically put into practice in the everyday job of treating patients; and even in our own times the problem of this time-lag has yet to be dealt with.

The work of Sydenham was taken up on the Continent by Boerhaeve, who was also paid the compliment of being called "a disciple of Hippocrates". He explored new paths by studying the changes that disease caused in the patient's organs after death and he illustrated the importance of this in excellent lectures to his students in the post-mortem room. From this stage, Morgagni progressed still further, examining the patient as far as was possible in sickness and in health, and drawing bold but logical conclusions regarding the full effect of illness on the afflicted person. He gave masterly descriptions of apoplexy, angina, syphilis, cirrhosis of the liver and many other ailments. Many text-book descriptions of diseases familiar to medical students were first put on medical record by Morgagni.

The extensive travel which characterised the Renaissance had one important result. A profusion of herbs and plants were discovered, and were classified scientifically by Linnaeus; so pharmacology and medical treatment gained by having a far wider range of drugs.

The advance in chemistry stimulated progress in the new science of physiology. Very little had been known about breathing and digestion, and now experimenters began to study what happened to food when it reached the stomach. Firstly, they demonstrated in the test-tube that food was digested by the gastric juices, and that the stomach muscles could not do the work alone without these important secretions. So digestion was not, after all, another form of putrefaction, which had been the accepted explanation. In the eighteenth century, Spallanzani confirmed these findings by a typically audacious experiment in which he swallowed bags and tubes which he studied after they had passed through his body.

Spallanzani performed many remarkable experiments, studying the smallest forms of life under the microscopes, and determined to arrive at the truth. He challenged the widely-held view that life could arise "spontaneously" from putrefying matter. Fertilisation demanded a male and a female component, he contended. He covered the male parts of frogs and toads with waxed linen during mating, and showed that the ova remained sterile: he then injected dog's sperm into a bitch, and procured artificial fertilisation. The older schools were loath to give up the centuries-old idea of "spontaneous generation", but Pasteur later gave the final death-blow to this concept.

A contemporary of Spallanzani, Haller (known as "the Great" even in his lifetime), is considered to be the founder of modern physiology. He carried out hundreds of original experiments and learned many new facts about breathing, digestion, the development of the embryo and many other mysteries. His most important work was on the function of the nervous system. Medical men thought that a fluid passed down the nerves to the muscles, and inflated them, so shortening them and making them contract. Haller demonstrated that muscles reacted to a stimulus which came through the nervous system. He correctly described the function of the central nervous system and its control over the whole body, but he thought that the vital element was the Soul, the living Principle.

Galvani and Volta applied theories of electricity to the body, and established that muscular contractions could be produced by electrical stimulation, but Volta proved that this was not a new form of electricity, impulsively named "Galvanism".

This better understanding of how the body was made and how it worked, in some ways complicated the task of the surgeon, but surgery became much more an exact science. Although the quality of surgical work continued to improve, no striking advance was made until the eighteenth century, when the great surgeon, John Hunter, raised surgery to the level of the other sciences. Hunter founded the methods of surgical pathology, and like most of the great scientists, was prepared to experiment on himself. On one occasion he accidentally innoculated himself with syphilis, but he turned the mishap into a good opportunity to study the disease at first-hand, and deliberately delayed treatment to do this. An accident to his ankle while dancing was used as a starting point for some useful research into the repair of torn tendons.

Hunter worked tirelessly to learn more about physiology: in particular, how structure determined function. He dissected and described more than 500 different types of animals, and did a great many experiments on repairing and transplanting injured tissues. His theory was not, however, as realistic as his practice, and he coined such meaningless phrases as "the irritation of imperfection" and "the blood's consciousness of being a useful part of the body", which classes him with the vague Vitalist philosophers. But when it came to the job in hand, he was always the bold scientist, as exemplified in his advice to Jenner, who showed hesitation about some practical work: "Don't think, try the experiment."

Medical theory in general moved forward with great strides in the first two centuries of the Renaissance. Doctors had acquired a much clearer picture of the body and its functions, and of the effect of disease on the body as a whole and on the different organs and connecting tissues that might be affected. Pathological study could therefore be directed to the most vital and significant aspects of the body, whether normal or diseased. Because of this comprehensive knowledge, the whole direction of medicine and surgery was profoundly influenced—at least, in theory. Practice, as usual, remained old-fashioned.

Bigwig and Near-Quack

It was a far cry from the exalted sphere of experiment and study to the crowded market place where medical treatment was sold like any other ware, or to the more refined atmosphere of the gilded drawing-room where, for an extravagant fee, the physician called when requested. Popular medicine of the seventeenth and eighteenth centuries was based on the occult and religious beliefs of the Middle Ages; only the outward appearance had changed a little.

In accordance with the well-established custom in all spheres of life, those who paid the most could command the best. Medical students, who themselves came from wealthy families, directed their ambitions towards serving the highest in the land, and their supreme aim was to become a court physician. Typical of the royal entourage was the medical household of Louis XII of France, which consisted of one Chief Physician and five assistants, five surgeons and assistants, two barbers, an apothecary and an astrologer. In contrast, the poor were left to the mercy of quacks and wise women.

The need for control was evident, and methods of licensing medical practitioners were introduced, but more to keep the circle small and select than to raise general standards. Thomas Linacre, physician to King Henry VIII, was empowered to set up a body of recognised physicians, which became the Royal College of Physicians; and they could decide who could practise in the City or within seven miles of it. About the same time, Thomas Vicary had Royal Assent to combine the guilds of surgeons and barber surgeons; and they had the power to inflict fines on offending practitioners.

Brilliant activities in all the sciences seemed in no way to penetrate the complacent dullness of most general practitioners. They covered their ignorance of the true nature of disease by impressive Latin phrases and technical jargon, and were hardly aware of the depth of their own ignorance. There was no clear distinction between physicians and the clan of charlatans, astrologers and necromancers who toured the land and sold their panaceas and secret remedies, with the skill and cunning of showmen; sometimes they were accompanied by a troupe of comedians who attracted customers by entertaining them with plays and sports.

The get-rich-quick atmosphere of the commercial world promoted an era of polished salesmanship in medicine. The ignorant public were not able to distinguish between the genuine marvels which science had discovered and the many false claims which were presented with eloquence and audacity by arrant quacks. Illiterate people were not alone in being duped: the self-styled "Count" Cagliostro gained the confidence of the highest circles, and sold his Waters of Youth and Elixir of Long Life even at the English Court. The English Government passed a special Act of Parliament to acquire Jane Steven's remedy for stone in the bladder, and she had made a large fortune before her "remedy" was finally examined and found to be made from useless substances. The general credulity of the public is illustrated in the common beliefs that blood-sucking vampires and hob-goblins caused epidemics, and that evil spirits entered the body and caused spasms and convulsive diseases.

In the eighteenth century Mesmer gained world-wide fame, and is not forgotten today. His theory was that every living body possesses a magnetic fluid exuding a special force which can make contact with other living bodies and the inorganic world. His practice was based on suggestion and hypnotism; his theatrical and dramatic methods bore some relation to primitive medicine, but his theories of "magnetic influences" had a mischievous effect on public credence. Variations on the patient-mesmerist relationship led to fantastic seances where anything but wholesome healing took place. Sometimes money was conjured out of people's pockets by the hypnotic power of clever sales-talk, such as that of Elisha Perkins who sold pairs of metal rods at five guineas a time, promising that they could extract disease when drawn downward over the affected part.

As a change from the long-cherished belief that if a sick person is given something of every drug, some good must come of it, Hahnemann introduced the theory of homoeopathy, the treatment of like with like. This teaching promoted an excellent reaction to the school prescribing many drugs; but in the prevailing atmosphere of uncritical acceptance of any new theory, it was soon being carried to absurd extremes. Hot compresses were applied to burns, opium given to somnolent patients, tapeworm heads given as medicine to people suffering from tapeworm, and gonorrhoea cases were treated with gonorrhoea pus.

Phrenology, another "science", was eagerly welcomed by a gullible public, and soon everyone was reading everyone else's bumps for signs of intellect and character.

These schools of medical practice were represented by the typical self-confident physician, swaggering in his dress of office, the square cap set firmly on the puffed-out wig, the long robe, and the impressive gold-mounted cane. During epidemics he wore the protective clothing fashionable in the Middle Ages, hiding behind a leather mask with glass-covered openings for the eyes, and sporting a long beak packed with antiseptics and perfumes. The wand with which he felt the patient's pulse might well have been the insignia of a witch-doctor. The bible of such physicians was *The London Pharmacopoeia*, the first edition of which appeared at the beginning of the seventeenth century; and its contents were worthy of the practitioners who used it. It contained about 2,000 remedies, including prescriptions of fox's lungs, oil of ants, oil of wolves, lozenges of dried vipers, and powders of precious stones. In the eighteenth century, revised editions introduced more rational remedies, such as digitalis and cinchona, a very useful tree-bark from which quinine was later derived. The old, popular traditions, however, would not be crowded out, and drugs such as essence of pearls, crayfish eye, and flesh of vipers were in constant use.

There was a continuous flow of new herbs and vegetables coming in with cargoes from all parts of the world, but they were not all of equal value, nor were they correctly assessed. When the potato first appeared, it was claimed as a cause of scrofula; tea and coffee were also suspected of causing nervous indispositions. Often, in practice, certain drugs were found to produce good results, but the way in which they worked was not understood correctly; for example, syphilis was treated with mercury because it was believed that the unhealthy matter was discharged in the extra flow of saliva, which mercury stimulated.

The Renaissance was a period of many conflicting trends in society. Expanding commerce encouraged men to be ambitious and astute, not least, the doctors. Medical practice, if it followed the popular tradition, could be an attractive proposition. What was the fashion in doctors? According to a criticism written a century later, "without at all understanding philosophy, mathematics, chemistry, or anatomy, without having studied diagnosis, symptomalogy, dietetics, or physiology, anyone can become a physician . . . it suffices for him to know by heart four aphorisms of Hippocrates, a dozen passages from Galen, and several other small quotations from a classical author, together with the names of various diseases, all of which could be included in one page of writing".

Like Aristophanes in the Greek period, Molière in the seventeenth century satirised in his play *Le Malade Imaginaire* the doctors who treated all his patients alike, with a mixture of old-fashioned remedies of enemas, purging and blood-letting, and cunning psychology. Such shafts go deep, but they take time to penetrate.

However, all abuses of science meet with their critics, and although the patent medicine drive was intensified with the wider use of newspaper advertisements, there were outspoken and courageous people who attacked the distortion of the true purpose of medicine. The monopoly of the Royal College of Physicians was also criticised, particularly the emphasis that was placed on income rather than need. In fact, the profession as a whole was accused of exploiting the ignorance of people and of using Latin to keep "trade secrets", for the purpose of filling its purse. There was no doubt that most physicians considered their main object and best interests to be caring for the wealthy; as was clearly demonstrated during the Great Plague, when even the more notable, including Sydenham, fled with their clients to the country.

The Royal College of Physicians established a dispensary in London, during the reign of James II, to provide free treatment for those whose poverty was certified by a clergyman; but the Apothecaries perceived in this a threat to their own interests, and by open opposition and in other ways, managed to bring the scheme to nothing. The jealousies and rivalries which flared up between various physicians did not help the practice of medicine or the cause of the patient, but the main obstacle to a wide advance was the general indifference to the adverse living and working conditions where ill health and disease were sown and spread.

However, as the period of the Renaissance moved onwards with ever growing cities and ports, men and machines becoming pressed ever harder in the service of commerce, some attention had to be paid to the ill effects of crowded and unhealthy conditions. Infectious diseases spread rapidly, and when the working ability of people was markedly affected, public health began to concern the owners of industry, who stimulated the authorities to take more effective action to keep the wheels turning. And so the science of public health was born.

Industry and Squalor

New worlds had opened up in the study of science and medicine, and great changes had taken place. What did they mean in terms of day-to-day life for the people?

The great change was, of course, the change-over from feudalism to the first stage of the industrial system. The people had always laboured for their daily bread; but the great difference now was in the volume of goods that flowed from working hands, applied more and more to machines and less and less to the plough. The increase of goods meant a swelling tide of wealth, which did not flow liberally over the land, nourishing all alike; it went in deep but narrow channels, for the benefit of the privileged class of merchants and factory owners. The mass of the people worked as they had always done; lived, ate, sickened and died as they had always done; and compelling the ungenerous authorities to concede at least the minimum of shelter and security.

During the Middle Ages the hamlets and villages had grown, in uneven and haphazard fashion, into thickly populated towns and ports. Plymouth, Manchester and Birmingham grew in importance; thousands of people evicted from the land through the Enclosures or cast adrift through the dissolution of the monasteries were drawn to the towns as the only places where they could find work. From the fifteenth century to the close of the reign of Queen Elizabeth, the population of England doubled until it was almost five millions.

The small wooden houses supported each other and often nearly met above the narrow, dark alleys which acted as open sewers for all the refuse from the rickety, rat-ridden homes. The sanitary arrangements were worse than primitive; city scavengers collected refuse from time to time and dumped their unpleasant loads outside the city walls, but, in the main, people lived in the midst of an accumulation of filth that might have sickened any savage transplanted suddenly from his simple village settlement into a "modern" industrial city. The London records about the time of the Great Plague give a typical case of what was quite usual in the way of housing: in one small house there lived eleven married couples and fifteen single persons. The basements and cellars of dwellings were often used as shops, workplaces and dairies. In an ill-directed effort to keep the population within manageable limits, the authorities often forbade the extension of the city, with the result that people living on the outskirts were even worse off, with no sanitary arrangements whatever for the dilapidated wooden sheds into which they all crowded, sharing all the horrors of civilisation and none of its amenities.

The plague and other infectious diseases made continuous assaults on the population, sweeping town and country with equal violence. The authorities had gained much experience in isolating nests of infection, and in disposing of the dead, but neither physicians nor politicians had yet grasped the fundamental concept of preventive medicine, namely, keeping people healthy by building up their defences against ill health.

The Great Fire of London in 1666 did more than any doctor or government to eradicate the septic conditions which bred infection among the people. Society was presented with a fine opportunity to rebuild London with a healthy regard for its citizens. Sir Christopher Wren had such visions of a well-planned city, but the main concern of the people who directed affairs was to return to "business as usual"; and so, with a few small improvements, the crowded tenements reappeared along the narrow streets, and the cesspits and sanitation remained as bad as before.

But no evils continue unchanged forever, although it may seem so to the generations who endure them. After the Plague and the Fire, streets were kept cleaner, and offensive trades came under closer regulations; by the end of the eighteenth century the townsfolk of London had pavements to walk along, and in France and America the installation of public baths brought them a little nearer to the hygiene of Ancient Rome.

In time, the people benefited by some of the up-to-date innovations which were introduced to help industrial production. For example, the water supply was improved after the introduction of steam pumps and iron pipes, although the streets in poor districts were supplied with only one tap and the quality of the water remained as tainted and as dangerous to health as before. On the other hand, the introduction of a window tax, designed to fill the national exchequer, reduced the nation's health by depriving people of light and sun in their homes and workplaces.

The prosperity of Britain was founded on its vast supplies of coal; the fires which drive British industry were lit during the Renaissance period. Forests of chimneys rose into the grey English skies: from soap-boiling factories to lime-burning kilns, from furnaces to the modest kitchen fire. And the smoke came down again to blacken everything from church to palace, and most harmful of all, the lungs of London's citizens. When Haydn visited London in 1791 he wrote in his diary: "A fog so thick that one might have spread it on bread; in order to write I had to light a candle as early as eleven o'clock", and Evelyn, the diarist, complained that Londoners were never free from coughs and almost one half of them died of "phthisical and pulmonic distempers"; his remedy was to plant large areas of sweet-smelling shrubs to mask the bad odours.

An important part of man's health is his diet. Most people during this period ate to live, and often scarcely managed that. The enjoyment of such choice luxuries as figs, apricots, sugar and sweets was the prerogative of the rich, and most people were fortunate if they obtained a regular supply of bare essentials. Nevertheless, the enclosing of so much arable land had directed attention to techniques of food-growing, promoting improvements in agricultural implements and in fertilising the soil. People learned to conserve cattle feeding-stuffs for the winter, so that there was an all-the-year round supply of fresh meat, butter and milk. Improved communications encouraged the bringing of more than the proverbial pig to market, and people were able to buy supplies of fresh vegetables in the lively centre of every small town.

Since water was suspiciously disease-producing, the last thing the people thought of doing was to drink it. Home-brewed ale was the popular thirst-quencher, and in the reign of Elizabeth it was discovered that the English soil was friendly to the growing of hops; and beer then became the working man's drink. In the year 1688, twelve million barrels of beer were brewed, for a population of five million. The Puritanical revulsion against excessive drinking had some justification from the health standpoint, in spite of Sir Toby Belch's rebuke to Malvolio, "Dost thou think, because thou art virtuous, there shall be no more cakes and ale?" But the situation grew more serious in the next century, when brandy was the drink of the nobility, rum for the middle classes, and gin for the poor. Gin-drinking was the main escape from the drab and hard life endured by most of the people. So much did drunkenness upset the working capacities and skills of the people, that the authorities were forced to pass several Gin Acts during the eighteenth century; but without much effect. The "pothouses" which had numbered one to every six dwelling places were at last banished to every street corner; but poverty, squalor and drunkenness remained inseparable; one could not be cured without the other.

The lack of sanitary conveniences, which lasted throughout the Middle Ages and well into the Renaissance, did not engender any enthusiasm for personal cleanliness among the general population. But gradually the understanding that health and cleanliness are associated produced some difference in the way of life of at least the upper class, who had the time and money to indulge in such luxuries. The fashion was set by Queen Elizabeth, of whom a newsletter reported: "The Queen doth bathe herself once a month whether she require it or not." The Queen and some of her Court had their own bathtubs, and had the exquisite pleasure of using scented soap; this, of course, was beyond the reach of the poor, who used wood-ashes, nettles, or even cow-dung to remove the surface dirt from their persons and their clothes.

The clothing worn did not make cleaning a simple matter. Articles like leather stays could never be washed, and stuffed and quilted petticoats were worn until they rotted; blankets remained on the bed until they became unusable. Later in the eighteenth century, cotton and calico came into use, and linen became cheaper and could be adapted to many purposes, including bed-covers, giving opportunities for improving considerably the standard of general hygiene of the people.

Unfortunately, the deplorable state of overcrowding and bad housing completely outweighed the small improvements in food and hygiene. Epidemic diseases were still the great undefeated, able at any time to strike down terrified populations, a grim challenge to the medical profession.

The Warfare of the Germs

The Middle Ages had known plague and pestilence, and against these terrible visitations humanity had struggled blindly, yet working industriously and laying the foundations of the Renaissance. The deplorable conditions did not improve greatly with the centuries, and infectious diseases were sown and spread wherever people lived and worked together in congestion and dirt.

The Renaissance was marked by a strange variation in the type and extent of the diseases which struck men down. There was a decline in leprosy and St Vitus's dance, and some lessening in the violent attacks of plague, but there was a large increase in measles, smallpox, typhus, influenza, tuberculosis, whooping-cough, scarlet fever, and in the low-lying places, malaria. It may be that there were better diagnosis and records in the later period; from all accounts it is clear that the people of the Renaissance faced many hazards from disease in the normal course of their life.

Of all the infectious diseases, plague spread the greatest terror throughout Europe, and it was most prevalent in the earlier centuries.

In the reigns of Henry VIII and Queen Elizabeth, tens of thousands died in London alone during epidemics. In the early seventeenth century, a million people died in Northern Italy during a four-year epidemic; and this terrible disease knew no frontiers. The Great Plague attacked London in 1665, and within seven months 100,000 people had been annihilated. By the end of the century, the populations of the capital cities of Austria and of those countries that now compose Czechoslovakia had filled mass graves in this losing battle with germs. After this, the fury of the onslaught began to slacken, but even so, in the first quarter of the eighteenth century it flared up again in parts of Europe as far distant as Russia and southern France, where the big ports of Marseilles and Toulon were the worst hit, with a death roll of almost 100,000 in one year alone.

In the general squalor and unhygienic way of life, bacteria jostled with each other for supremacy over the miserable suffering mass of humanity which was their happy hunting ground. From the fifteenth to the sixteenth centuries, a now obsolete disease known as the sweating sickness—a brief but horrible attack lasting only twenty-four hours —killed thousands of people. Smallpox raged throughout this period, and has not yet been defeated in every part of the world, although science has now found the means of victory which were unknown in Tudor England, when the Sovereign, Queen Mary herself, succumbed to the disease. Smallpox became more virulent as the centuries passed, and at the beginning of the eighteenth century 14,000 died in Paris in one year alone, and at the end of the century, three million in India. Infants and young people fell the easiest victims, and smallpox became known, with a bitter cynicism, as "the friend of the poor man who happens to be burdened with a large family".

Amongst this band of marauders, typhus was well to the front, particularly among populations most reduced by famine and poverty. Lice carried the typhus germ to the very places where people were most subject to dirt, neglect and overcrowding, and so typhus had many aliases: gaol-fever, ship-fever, hospital and putrid fever. This disease was no respecter of persons, and when the opportunity presented, it spread from the lowly criminal in the dock to the exalted judge on the bench; as happened in 1577 at Oxford where the typhus germ passed sentence of death on the entire court, the two justices, the county sheriff and the whole of the grand jury, and then on many citizens of the town.

Conditions of war were particularly encouraging to typhus; and during the frequent battles that engaged the armies of Italy, Spain and the Low Countries, each army had to contend with the invisible enemy that attacked both sides; in the same way, England suffered during the period of the Civil War, particularly at the sieges of Oxford and Reading, among populations weakened by bloodshed and hunger.

Typhus spread continuously in the ever more congested towns, and especially in times of widespread undernourishment caused through bad harvests. In the beginning of the eighteenth century London suffered three outbreaks, the last killing more than one tenth of the population; the poor suffered the greatest hardship and losses, but no door, even those of the wealthy, could be effectively locked and barred against the entry of disease.

One of the most frightening diseases, previously unknown, appeared with the growth of civilisation. Syphilis was the unwelcome visitor, and "the other country" was consistently blamed for its arrival. It had been named the "French" and "Neapolitan" disease, the "Spanish complaint" and, internationally, the "pox"; the theory that it had been brought from the Americas with the homecoming crew of Christopher Columbus is probably false. The disease assailed people during the late medieval period, and was often confused with leprosy; there is direct evidence that an epidemic occurred among the troops in the French invasion of Italy in 1494; wherever it appeared, it inflicted great loss of life. It was only later that its venereal origin was recognised; and it became associated, in a similar manner, with the abhorrence that was aroused by leprosy; an attitude of mind which did not help towards rational treatment.

These were the outstanding enemies of the people, but many other germs sometimes unidentified by the doctors could also claim overwhelming victories; tuberculosis was recognised only in its final stage; and although the people suffered from diphtheria, measles, scarlet fever and typhoid fever, these diseases were often confused with one another; the miseries of the common people were often nameless and countless.

Paradoxically, physicians directed their main attention to treating their paying patients, who did not suffer to the same extent from infectious diseases. This carefully protected little world appeared to be all that concerned those who moved within its circle. A physician practising among the rich wrote in 1784: "There has been but one instance of a truly malignant fever happening in the town for many years." Clearly he had never discussed medical affairs with a colleague, Dr Currie, who at the same time was seeing about 160 sick cases every week at his dispensary. But for every quietly devoted Dr Currie, there were many whose activities were circumscribed by their own narrow interests.

Medical Counter-attacks

There had to be an organised strategy to defeat these diseases which had for so long plagued unprotected mankind. Other sciences had advanced from the first methodical steps of collecting facts and data; infectious diseases were first studied in a similar scientific manner by John Graunt in the seventeenth century. His book *Natural and Political Observations upon the Bills of Mortality* was followed by the work of Sir William Petty, now revered as "the Father of Political Economy", who published his important *Essays on Political Arithmetic*. This work dealt with the population death-rate and disease figures, and gave the history of an epidemic and the effect achieved by medical intervention. Petty demonstrated what individual industrialists had already concluded—industry as a whole was the loser by the great sickness and death rates amongst the workers. He suggested that the Government should be concerned with the health of its most productive members, the farmers, manufacturers, merchants and seamen. This work was of great value, but it did not deal with the next most important question in the battle: how epidemic disease originated.

Epidemic diseases were more than a question of life and death for the individual; it was evident that the relations between people were as complex as the means of production, and any form of breakdown affected the whole life of the community. With an energy born of necessity, a new drive was made against these socially disabling diseases.

Quarantine and destruction of infected goods impeded the commercial interests whose laden ships were coming in a continuous stream to every port of call. Perhaps the real source of infection could be sought elsewhere: in bad smells, cesspits and stagnant waters which abounded? Could the spread of disease be stopped by early notification of the first cases and their removal to so-called "houses of recovery"? Possibly fumigation and disinfection would kill the disease without its being necessary to destroy the valuable goods in which it was supposed to be lurking?

The authorities were persuaded to direct their attention along these lines, and so the foundation of sanitary reform was laid down. The Lords of the Regency appointed a special physician, Dr Mead, in 1719, to guide the Government in the best way to deal with the plague; he recommended the employment of "searchers" for the dead and skilled physicians for the sick; prompt isolation of infected patients and the disinfection of people and houses; he also advised notification.

The Missing Clue

From medieval times, men had grappled with epidemic diseases. Sometimes they had come close to the fundamental cause by experiment and logic; but without the aid of the microscope they could not come to grips with the actual culprit, the invisible microbe.

The great search continued. Clearly, outbreaks stemmed mainly from the crowded and dirty parts of cities, so a drive was developed to clean up the noisome lanes and passages; orders went out to sweep streets, to keep gutters clean and sweet-smelling; and scavengers, the forerunners of sanitary inspectors, were appointed to carry out the work. Animals came under suspicion as possible carriers of plague and immediately a great campaign was under way to keep down the swarms of vermin and small animals like cats and swine. During the Great Plague special officers were employed to kill and bury stray dogs, and 40,000 were destroyed in a short time. Unfortunately, the greatest criminal, the rat, was thought to be of little importance; after both the epidemic and the panic had died down, he was left to run freely in the heaps of dirt which soon returned after the new broom of authority, which had swept so clean, was allowed to rest again in a dusty corner. The rat scampered around the dung-heaps and in and out of the verminous homes of the poor; and the germs of disease smouldered unchecked, ready to flare up again in man at the first opportunity.

However, as early as the sixteenth century, Fracastoro outlined a rational theory of contagion. He reasoned that infectious diseases could be passed on in three ways: by simple contact, as in scabies and leprosy; by indirect contact, through such things as bedclothes which, although not affected themselves, could carry the seeds of the disease and so pass it from one person to another; and the third means of transmission, over a distance, he surmised by observing the spread of plague and smallpox; the disease in some form must pass through the air, and so he argued that infection must be the result of the spread of minute bodies which could propagate unceasingly.

By this reasoning, Fracastoro came closer to the theory of germs than did any one else during the next two centuries. The great importance of his teaching was that it determined the most effective forms of action against spreading epidemics—isolation and disinfection. Medieval customs were carried on with even greater rigour. The population were warned of the presence of plague and pestilence in the traditional ways; throughout the Renaissance the leper's bell rang, and the front doors of afflicted homes carried the dreaded sign of the red cross and the words "Lord have mercy upon us", as they had done for the previous 200 years. The searchers who undertook their unsavoury job came as always from the roughest and most needy people, and many cruel and corrupt deeds were practised on the helpless families who fell into their hands.

Where were the people of authority who normally kept tolerable order in the affairs of the city? During these epidemics, not only public and private business but the Law Courts and Parliament itself were hastily suspended; and the officials and all who could afford the expense, speedily removed themselves to the country, as far from danger as possible. People were forbidden to gather together in any number, and on saints' days beggars were excluded from the churches to avoid bringing in contagion. In 1563, when Queen Elizabeth returned for safety to Windsor, gallows were set up in the market place "to hang all such as should come from London".

There were those who fell ill and died or struggled back to health within their own four walls; but something had to be done about the many vagrant and homeless people, who most frequently were the earliest victims of infection. The order went out that "small tents or cabins made of a few boards and such materials as may soonest be put together" were to be erected in the interests rather of the uncontaminated than of the sick. These small pest-houses, which undoubtedly lived down to their name, were nevertheless the forerunners of our modern isolation hospitals.

However, not all accepted Fracastoro's views and the prescribed methods of combating contagion. Without respite, people were haunted with a grim fear; they had to find some answer to disease. If medical men were helpless to prevent it, then there must be some witchcraft in it; fear and ignorance drove people to terrible deeds. During the sixteenth and seventeenth centuries hundreds of thousands of "witches" were hunted out, accused of having cast evil spells for spreading infectious diseases; such an accusation signified death at the stake: there was no escape. Protestant and Catholic countries alike were guilty of extracting confessions to these "crimes" by means of torture to which only death brought relief.

If doctors could not stop contagious diseases, still less could they cure them. Any form of remedy was tried, from charms and amulets to dried toad powder, a "true philosophical preparation of potable gold", and the Royal College of Physicians' Plague Water, which had twenty-one ingredients.

The battle against the unknown germs was waged on the Continent on similar rational and irrational lines. Doctors practising rational medicine in the hot and marshy lands of Italy suggested that stagnant waters and swamps should be drained, and sanitary guards stationed in large cities to demand certificates of health from incoming travellers.

Other infectious diseases were tackled in the same spirit. Tuberculosis received particular attention, although for so many centuries it had, almost unchallenged, killed countless numbers. Fracastoro had recognised how difficult a disease it was to combat. He had written: "If it were possible to destroy [the germs of the disease in the lungs] by the use of caustics, there would be no better remedy; but because such remedies cannot be employed without danger to the organ, it is necessary to treat them through adjacent organs." Doctors in

England and on the Continent could not track down the cause of the disease, but experience had already taught the effectiveness of taking precautions to safeguard others. Clothing and linen were fumigated, sputum was disinfected, and patients were isolated in hospitals specially built for them.

It was a to-and-fro battle. Some diseases, like malaria, were indirectly brought under control through improving sanitation and draining swampy land required for agriculture and industrial developments. Others, like scarlet fever, influenza, measles and whooping-cough proved too much for all efforts; indeed this is not surprising, as we know very little even today of the way in which these diseases are spread.

In about the 1760's, there was a suggestion of a clue that typhoid had some connection with contaminated well-water; but the common belief was that the culprit who poisoned the wells was that centuries-old scapegoat, the Jew.

From the time that syphilis made its appearance, great efforts were made to overcome it; in the first confusion and panic, it was thought to be due to some evil conjunction of the planets, or to misdeeds of the victim; but gradually more rational thinking decided on treatment and isolation. Methods were often harsh, and sufferers were sometimes expelled from the towns, as in Paris, or isolated in the special houses once reserved for lepers. Prostitutes were banished, whipped and branded, but more humane treatment gradually replaced the early brutalities, which arose from a mixture of fear and moral condemnation. In Germany and Italy, hospitals were established for syphilitics; and in this disease as with all others, the rational treatment began to win good results.

Many of the contagious diseases caused great suffering and death, but the one most hated was the disfiguring smallpox, which left its ugly mark on the face of every victim who survived an attack. So common was it that a woman of the eighteenth century was considered beautiful merely if she possessed a smooth, unpitted skin.

The possibility of inoculation against this disease had been known from primitive times; the ancient Chinese had practised it, and with commendable initiative, Lady Mary Wortley Montagu, wife of the British Ambassador to Turkey, encouraged its use in England in the early part of the eighteenth century. But the really conclusive experiment was undertaken by Jenner, who was put on to the trail of vaccination by a chance remark he overheard from a dairymaid who said: "I cannot take smallpox, for I have had cowpox." Encouraged by his teacher, John Hunter, Jenner dared to try the experiment, and in truly scientific spirit tested it in every possible way, until he established a landmark in medical history by proving that an epidemic disease could to some extent be brought under control. Even today, there are people who strongly oppose vaccination, but the fact remains that through its practice a hideous and death-dealing disease has become comparatively rare, and human happiness has increased accordingly.

Slowly but steadily the gradual improvement in general hygiene and medical knowledge helped to make headway against difficulties that had at one time seemed insurmountable.

More Gains by Medicine and Science

The northern isles were sending their ships and goods everywhere over the high seas; but ships and guns had to be manned, and long sea journeys in relatively light craft called for strength and stamina, in a word—health.

Many crews set out from England on these venturesome voyages, and before they had sailed many days, men were struck down by the same fever that overwhelmed thousands in the armed forces and in prisons. Typhus and scurvy were threatening to rob England of the wealth and power which promised to place her ahead of all other nations.

The outstanding medical men of the eighteenth century, Lind, Sir Gilbert Blaine, Pringle, and Howard, sponsored the campaign for better health and so contributed to the success of their rising century.

Lind investigated the general conditions of sailors. He found that they lived and worked, as it were, in a floating slum. In stormy weather there was no ventilation at all for the men below-decks; only the senior officers had cabins offering reasonable light or space. The food was of the worst quality, mainly biscuits, half-salted beef which was often putrid and one pint of water a day per man for all needs, including drinking. Lind saw that in such cramped conditions disease was bound to spread through dirty and infected clothing, especially as many of the crews came straight from prison to the ships. He campaigned for better conditions, and in particular recommended an improved diet, including fruit juices, which he maintained would prevent scurvy.

The painful affliction of scurvy attacked the seafaring peoples of Northern Europe. In all the famous voyages of the time which made nautical and geographical history, men were laid low and killed by this inexplicable scourge. Admiral Hawkins estimated that he had lost 10,000 men from scurvy in twenty years of sea-going, and in the early eighteenth century Lord Anson lost more than three-quarters of his men on a four-year journey round the world. Various explanations were given: change of air, a weak stomach, and a "scorbutic constitution", before Lind emphasised the importance of a balanced diet including fresh fruit and vegetables.

Then came the famous experiment of Captain Cook. On his travels in the South Seas, in a journey lasting over three and a half years, he did not lose a single man, a result obtained by the simple method of adding lemon juice to the rations. It took twenty-five years for the Government to learn the lesson, but after further pressure from medical quarters, and the deplorable occurrence of over 2,000 cases affecting the Channel Fleet after a ten-weeks' cruise, the machinery began at last to move. At the end of the eighteenth century, an Admiralty Order required that lemon juice should be used on board. From that time, scurvy was banished from British ships.

Pringle took up the cudgels on behalf of the army. His work on military hygiene, *Observations on Diseases of the Army*, was a bestseller, running into seven editions. As a result of his recommendations, army serving conditions were revolutionised. The men were provided with suitable clothing, good boots, well-planned sanitation and drainage, and proper ventilation in the sleeping quarters; adequate food, rest and exercise all helped to reduce infection and sustain morale.

The authorities soon recognised the importance of environment, as expounded by a contemporary of Pringle, Sir Gilbert Blaine, who said: "The means of prevention are more within our power than those of cure; for it is more in human art to remove contagion, to alter man's food and clothing, to command what exercises he is to use, and what air he is to breathe, than it is to produce any given change in the internal operation of the body."

Nevertheless, uncomfortable and unhygienic conditions were the rule, and the prisons were, not unexpectedly, the worst in dirt and neglect. The bad conditions outside, and the general struggle to keep going in the rush and tumble of a competitive world, drove more and more people downwards, many landing eventually in over-crowded gaols. A newcomer to the criminal population found himself locked in a small room, from nine in the morning until five the next morning, with thirty or even forty other wretched people, men, women and children. Sanitary arrangements consisted of one privy, and there was neither bed nor cover. The clean and the verminous lay down together, and it did not take very long for infected lice to carry typhus throughout the prison. People in authority showed signs of alarm when, somewhat late in the day, they began to see that prison bars were not a cage for disease. In the Easter Session of the Old Bailey, in 1750, the Lord Mayor and other important persons died from the same contagion that was raging in Newgate Prison. Inquiry revealed that "the whole prison of Newgate and all the passages leading thence were in a very filthy condition and had long been so".

At last the ground was ready for the seed sown by the social reformer and hygienist. Howard was well aware of these appalling conditions in prisons both in England and abroad. He had studied the whole question thoroughly, and he recommended that patients should be separated from healthy prisoners, baths should be available, and clothes baked as a means of destroying infection. He insisted that a sick person, whether he was a convicted criminal or no, should have the help of a physician and apothecary. Howard declared that these measures would save many more lives than all the medicines in the apothecaries' shops.

Bitter experience, and the work of such people as Howard, at last persuaded those who were in a position to introduce some preventive measures; the wealthy themselves began to choose more hygienic and comfortable living quarters, and by the end of the eighteenth century typhus had scored its last major victory in England. The

method of experimenting and learning from practice, even without
a basic understanding of the cause of the trouble, was bringing encouraging results.

What had been done in tackling typhus, smallpox and scurvy
could possibly be applied to other ailments. Doctors with a scientific
outlook turned to other mystifying complaints. There was, for example, that trouble, Devonshire colic, associated with drinking cider.
Between September, 1762, and July, 1767, almost 300 cases had been
taken into Exeter hospitals. What was happening in Devon that
apparently did not occur elsewhere? Sir George Baker noticed that
the symptoms were similar to those shown by painters who suffered
from lead-poisoning. Having this clue, chemical analysis showed that
Devonshire cider contained lead,—from the lead lining of the cider
presses, a type used only in Devon.

And so finally the scientific method was established for medicine.
It was a long step forward from alchemy and astrology, which had
been the principal means of deduction for thousands of years; it was
a step that had taken only 200 years; and now a long road, but the
right road for medical science, stretched ahead.

The State Shows an Interest in Health

From the beginning of the Middle Ages, a few hospitals had been
established, and some doctors had been officially appointed to cope
with the numbers of sick people who would otherwise have died in
the streets, spreading contagion unchecked. As cities and industries
grew, and with them complicated problems of living and widespread
poverty, new illnesses threatened society as a whole.

The number of doctors appointed to organise the necessary services had to be continuously increased. Acting as coroners and police
surgeons, supervising private practitioners and public health regulations, and in their spare time treating the poorest patients free, and
others according to a sliding scale, these found their hands full. There
were other duties connected with the supervision of ships, watering
places, and of course the pressure of relentless epidemics to be faced.

By the end of the eighteenth century, the work had grown too
much for one man, or even for a number of men, working singly.
The first dispensaries for the sick were established in London in 1770,

and gloomy and forbidding though they were, there was an immediate flow of patients from the poverty-stricken slums in the midst of which they had been built.

The old pest-houses and isolation places of the Middle Ages, and the few charitable institutions initiated by the monks, set the pattern for the general hospitals; but in spite of the obvious need, very little was done in the seventeenth century except for the building of Greenwich Hospital for wounded and disabled seamen. Slowly, at intervals of decades, fever hospitals were built, first in Manchester, then in London and Liverpool; but always the number of sick people was far greater than the number of beds available.

Hospitals had been established, but what were they like? Howard, who had directed his criticism against the spread of typhus in prisons, probed with equal courage into the question of hospitals. Howard challenged municipal complacency with his public descriptions of those he visited. Famous hospitals were exposed for being generally dirty, neglected, and, worst of all, for their verminous and unhealthy conditions. St Thomas's had no water-closets; in Middlesex Hospital, patients lay in wooden beds enclosed by suffocating hangings, and the air breathed by the sick was even worse than that circulating in the wards. The staff were untrained, badly fed and poorly paid. Hospitals were in fact a breeding-ground for disease; cruelty, drunkenness and immorality among the staff were commonplace. Howard's indictment helped to bring about some rebuilding and improvements, but even at the end of the century, patients on entering hospital still had to pay deposits to cover possible funeral expenses.

Despite the dread they aroused, hospitals were always crowded, because working conditions in factories were not organised to protect health. On the contrary, machines were set up and workers herded into any available shed or cellar; the only concern was to satisfy the clamour coming from all over the world for English goods.

Industrial diseases were nothing new, but the workers' burden of suffering as a result of their labours was unequalled in history. Thousands of workers using lead suffered from paralysis; mercury vapour poisoned many in a variety of trades, including gold refiners, glassmakers, and felt-makers stooping long hours over steam kettles; bakers and textile workers succumbed to many complaints caused by overheated and dusty workrooms; Birmingham metal-workers contracted alarming symptoms of green hair and red eyes; and to supply essential power to all these industries, the miners toiled incessantly in hastily sunk pits, unprotected against the constant threat of accident and death.

These conditions were crying out for attention from doctors. Here was a new sphere of study, and the first scientific survey of industrial diseases was made by Ramazzini, who, in 1700 published a famous book, *The Diseases of artificers, which by their particular callings they are most liable to, with the Method of avoiding them, and their Cure.* Originally written in Italian, this book was translated into English fifty years later.

Ramazzini considered a wide variety of occupations, from leather workers to athletes. Like investigators in other spheres, he concluded that with a general improvement in diet and less arduous work, people would be able far more effectively to resist attacks on their health. His concluding words have importance for all times: "Pecuniary gain is worthless if it entails the loss of what is best worth having, health ... we owe this to the wretched condition of the workers from whose manual toil, so necessary though sometimes mean and sordid, so many benefits accrue to the commonwealth of mankind; yes, this debt must be paid by the most glorious of all arts (as Hippocrates calls it in his Precepts) that of Medicine, which cures without a fee and succours the poor."

Further studies by Thackrah showed that in Great Britain, at least 50,000 people died each year through external influences of home and workplace. He, too, was moved not only by scientific curiosity, but by feelings of indignation at the unnecessary suffering caused by preventable conditions. Thackrah developed the method of studying a special area, Leeds, and comparing the effect of environment on the death rate; he demonstrated how health could be affected by the section of the city in which a person lived, as well as by such disturbing influences as low, fluctuating wages, accidents, deformities and intemperance.

Mothers and Children

Infant life was held cheap in the eighteenth century. All the discomforts and sickness that struck at the adult population had a deadly effect on the young. Up to the middle of the eighteenth century the average mortality was four out of every ten babies born alive; and seven out of every ten died before their fifth birthday. Sickness alone could not have produced this mass murder; it was aided and abetted by social conditions which compelled parents to abandon and expose great numbers of infants when they had not the means to rear them.

Once again, medical knowledge and authority had to work together to overcome an outstanding social evil. In the middle of the eighteenth century a Foundling Hospital was established to receive abandoned children, and thirty years later the Government passed an Act which enabled children dependent on the parish to be cared for. Although these measures, together with improvements in the knowledge of child welfare, helped to reduce death rates by one-half, the future of these rescued children was by no means a happy one. Their childhood came to an end from the age of five or six, when most of them were sent into the grim factories of the Midlands, there to serve a hard-driven apprenticeship which illness and death frequently interrupted before the age of fourteen.

Even the children who received a naturally loving welcome into the heart of their families were almost smothered out of existence by too many swaddling clothes and too little fresh air and clean water. The prevailing old-wives' tales proclaimed that clean clothing would deprive babies of their natural juices, that cow's milk to drink would give a child cowlike characteristics, and that a poultice-like mess of bread-and-water was the proper diet after breast-feeding. As a result, rickets was common, bandy legs seemed inevitable, and a general lowering of resistance made the child open to every roaming infection.

Wet-nursing was popular among the rich, who, like the poor, had large families but could find more convenient means of shedding their responsibilities. Wet-nurses were generally untrained and ignorant, and although infants could not tell of the ill-treatment they received at lazy and brutal hands, some physicians became aware of the evil consequences of careless farming-out of children and tried to teach sensible child care and regular feeding habits. As for the children of the poor, even tender and loving parents were compelled to apprentice them at the age of six or seven years; and as these children often lived and slept at their place of work, there was every likelihood that they would never return.

To give birth to a child in these times was a hazard as dangerous as working in the mines. The great danger to mothers was child-bed fever, which nullified the advantages gained from the establishment of maternity hospitals in the middle of the eighteenth century. Doctors had made some improvements in conducting confinements, by removing the task of delivering the baby from the dirty and clumsy hands of superstitious midwives. As early as the sixteenth century, Dr Peter Chamberlen invented the forceps, which, however, was kept as a family secret for 125 years, before its use was learnt and modified by the skilled obstetricians William Smellie and William Hunter, the brother of the famous John Hunter.

Nobody knew of the existence of germs, but there had been ample demonstrations of the effectiveness of cleanliness in keeping disease at bay. Up-to-date surgeons like Dr White and Dr Smellie practised care and cleanliness in handling all their cases. Dr Smellie advised that forceps should not be used too often; in fact, forceps were a common cause of child-bed fever because of the lack of aseptic precautions; Dr White proudly claimed that he had never lost a mother from child-bed fever.

The results of applying the best knowledge of that time was summed up in the *Medical Memoirs* of Dr Lettson, who wrote at the end of the eighteenth century: "In the nurture and management of infants, as well as in the treatment of lying-in women, the reformation hath equalled that in the smallpox. By these two circumstances alone incredible numbers have been rescued from the grave."

The Advance from the Fifteenth to the Eighteenth Century

The Renaissance had opened with the sudden bursting of many bonds. Old forms of living, old ways of producing the bread of life, and the old narrow confines of travel and commerce, had been broken through, and a new social order had emerged. The eyes of science had opened wide and looked round at the real world. Medicine, too, had found the incentive and the conditions in which it could shed the old habits and take on new forms.

By the end of the eighteenth century, the first tentative moves towards the State's accepting responsibility for dealing with ill-health had crystallised into a clearly defined function. The foundation of modern public health and hygiene was laid down by Frank in a four-volume treatise, *A Complete System of Medical Policy*.

He described a very comprehensive field of public health protection, ranging from proper drainage, school hygiene and meals for children, to a proposed tax on bachelors. He introduced the idea of a trained body of "medical police". He also had the honour to be the first to propose family allowances, so that children should not suffer through the poverty of their parents.

At the same time, an American reformer, Count Rumford of Massachusetts, was campaigning in his country for better public hygiene. He advocated improving the conditions of the poor, lowering the cost of living, and providing inexpensive and healthy homes with cheap supply of heat and light, warm meals for school children and soup kitchens for the hungry.

The investigations of scurvy had drawn attention to the general need for improving diet and replacing excessive drinking of spirits by more varied supplies of vegetables and fruit, and by less harmful drinks such as tea and coffee.

Nevertheless, the general run of doctors and physicians carried on in the old way, treating the wealthy with consideration, and the poor with that lack of enthusiasm which the chilly atmosphere of charity seems to engender. But forward-looking medical men were already teaching that the key to good health lay in the study of a man's whole life, particularly of his working conditions.

Necessity had already brought about some action by the State on behalf of the people. The foundations of the scientific medicine of the future had been laid at the close of the Renaissance. The swiftly-changing conditions that lay ahead were to bring great new problems to the science of medicine—and the challenge was accepted.

Chapter Seven

THE INDUSTRIAL REVOLUTION (1)

Steam and Steel

FOR England and Wales the nineteenth century opened resoundingly. The increasing clangour of industrial activity had been growing since the first creakings of wooden machinery replaced the hand-power of craftsmen in the previous century. The momentous discovery of the power of steam was a godsend to the ambitious factory-owner, who was now no longer dependent on the wayward water-power of the valleys. Factories sprang up where labour was most plentiful and markets nearest to hand.

Textiles and woollen goods were the principal output of the ever-hungry machinery, which raw materials and human toil fed night and day, and the clatter of the flying shuttles of England began to sound across the world. There was a world of potential customers, and what could not be paid for in money could be more than amply repaid in raw materials and the native products so attractive to those who had the cash necessary for imported luxuries.

Most satisfying of all, the British producers were well ahead of other Western countries; at the beginning of the nineteenth century, England could claim to be the first to enter the race for turning out cheap, mass-produced goods, first in the field with the necessary technical and scientific equipment, first in creating an industrialised population trained and organised to work at the highest pitch— and first in possessing the largest and most congested of industrial towns.

Man's laboured progress through the long ages of bronze and iron had brought him, with an unexpected suddenness, into a new age— the age of steel and electricity. These gigantic sources of power charged the sluggish movement of history with dynamic energy. The merchants of capital, already the ruling power in the most civilised nations, eagerly harnessed these imposing tools to the rapidly expanding productive forces, in their ceaseless effort to command the

markets of the world. Steam navigation, railways and electric telegraph were developed with striking speed and skill; time and distance
were brought under man's control; there was no breathing-space left
to wonder. In all spheres of activity, the headlong rush was on: to
turn out more and yet more goods, to sell farther and yet farther
afield, to accumulate greater and greater wealth. This, however, was
possible only for the few who owned the means to get ahead in the
scramble; for the many there were the mill, the mine, and the growing competition for the job of serving the menacing machines; living
and working was geared to a higher speed than man had ever known
before.

New Worlds for Science to Conquer

Scientific knowledge helped to speed the general tempo. Commercial interests pressed impatiently for solutions to the many problems which emerged from the increasingly complex machines and
methods of production and distribution. The different sciences, particularly chemistry, were brought into the struggle to overcome
practical difficulties. The problems facing industry stretched across a
wide front. There was the growing army of workers who had to
be fed; and if the processes of nature were too slow, they must be
speeded up. Since textiles must be made ever more attractive in a
competitive trade, new dyes and colour combinations had to be found
to tempt the market. Steam and electricity were unruly servants, so
the experts must help to tame them and drive them along ever new
paths. All the specialists were called upon, but the chemist was given
the most urgent problems to solve with his test-tubes and his revealing microscope.

Chemistry made a spectacular advance in dealing with problems
of agriculture, dyeing processes, and in particular the specific problems of the silk and wine industries. Even in the medical world, the
man of the age was undoubtedly Pasteur—a chemist, not a doctor.
The profoundly important discovery that living organisms were the
cause of many diseases was made, indirectly, by Pasteur. Both the
silk and the wine trades had been afflicted by a sudden deterioration
in their products, and in desperation the manufacturers sought technical advice and help. Pasteur studied the subject in the field; an

entire industry depended on the results of his observations and the laboratory tests. Pasteur solved the riddle for the business world, and in so doing, he helped to change the whole future of medicine.

In other times, such remarkable advances would have taken months and even years before they were common knowledge; but now the printed word could be flashed across the world. A scientist could board a train in Berlin or Moscow and quickly arrive in Paris to see for himself the new experiments which from afar had aroused his curiosity.

With all these modern aids, scientists were able to work as a body, each contributing in some measure to the general forward movement.

Many important additions to knowledge were made by this concerted action. At last the true nature of breathing was analysed by Lavoisier, who demonstrated that oxygen was taken in through the lungs, and the unwanted carbon dioxide and water vapour breathed out after chemical changes had taken place in the living laboratory of the body; soon it was shown that the vital changes took place in the tissues and not in the blood. Then came the solution to one of the most baffling problems of all times: what was the source of the animal heat and power that kept living things alive? Helmholtz, experimenting with chemical changes that produce heat, discovered that all forms of energy—heat, light, electricity, motion and all chemical reactions—can be changed from one to another, and he demonstrated that energy could neither be created nor destroyed. This was a reality more wonderful than the medieval dream of the philosopher's stone for changing base metal into gold.

A New Science: the Study of Life

The exciting advances in this most recent science threw new light on the mysteries of the human body. It had taken hundreds of years to build up a reasonably accurate picture of the frame and structure of a man. But in the century of the great industrial revolution it became possible for medicine to leap forward into an entirely new and revolutionary branch of knowledge: the intimate study of living matter, the science of biology.

It was known that organic life is subject to chemical changes, some of which could be demonstrated in the laboratory. From this basis, a hundred and one exciting clues were followed to trace the origin of the body's functions.

It became clear that the processes of digestion and assimilation of food could be explained by chemical action. Chemicals that were found in the body could be made synthetically in the laboratory. This encouraged a deeper study of the chemical reactions of all parts of the body, and an important discovery was made that would have astonished the Greeks, who had taught that heat was one of the four inherent attributes of the body. Now the chemists learned that the body's heat was produced as a result of the combustion of food.

Food, and the soil from which it grew, could be analysed chemically; and it was seen that living things were composed of chemical compounds reacting with others, breaking them down and building them up again. Such an intense concentration on chemical analysis inevitably led some scientists to a one-sided view of natural processes; for example, they firmly held that fermentation was the operation of chemical changes only, and this seemed logical enough until Pasteur detected that the changes resulted from the activities of living germs.

In France, a great physiologist, Claude Bernard, carried the new knowledge into experimental work in medicine. He worked in the true manner of the pioneers of science, as he described in his own advice to his colleagues: "Put off your imagination as you do your overcoat when you enter the laboratory . . . lest it hinder your observing power . . . but before the experiment and between whiles, let your imagination wrap you round."

Bernard learned new facts about the chemical action of the bodily organs, in particular, the work performed by the liver in storing sugar, which it changed into a convenient form, glycogen, ready for the body's needs. He carried out biochemical experiments and found he could produce disease artificially with the use of chemicals; by reversing the process, he used chemicals for treating disease and laid the foundation for the scientific study of drugs.

He also forecast the modern approach to bodily disorders: illness as a reaction of the body to an adverse external environment. He suggested that the body has its own internal environment controlled mainly by changes in the blood which circulated through all the tissues. Health depended upon the harmonious working together of all parts of the body, which could be upset by serious changes in the external environment. This teaching was in direct contrast to the view of disease as being located in one special organ or part of the body; the value of the new approach was that it laid emphasis on the need to control the factors which affect people and their general well-being.

Powerful support for the theory of the influence of environment on living beings came with the dramatic publication of the life-work of Charles Darwin, *The Origin of Species*. Within the pages of this scholarly study he built up an incontestable case against the ancient myths on the nature of life, its unchanging and unchangeable character and the sudden creation of man and animals a mere few thousand years ago. Darwin demonstrated that man was linked by common bonds to all other living creatures with whom he had shared the world for millions of years. He unfolded an exciting history of great varieties and forms of life struggling against difficulties and learning to adapt and change, and even to evolve into new species, with the survival of the fittest flowering into the most noble of all creatures, thinking, feeling, man.

Darwin, Bernard, Pasteur and many other scientists of the age were making the most positive contributions yet achieved in the great story of evolution. By transforming medicine into a science, they were developing man's power to control nature, and to work consciously for an environment which would help man to reach his full stature.

The more the biologists and physiologists studied, the more they found there was to learn about the intricate make-up and working of the body. The mysteries of the central nervous system challenged the attention of the investigators. How did the brain send the command to the feet: "Forward march!"? How did the feet let the brain know, "We're tired!"? Even more intriguing was the problem: how did the body defend itself by sneezing, coughing or blinking, with no conscious awareness of what was going on?

The brain was found to be the centre of bodily control, receiving and sending messages to all parts of the body, including the sense organs, through the many nerves, which radiated like telephone wires from the brain and spinal cord.

The discovery of electrical reactions inspired experiments with the nervous system. What would happen if an electrical stimulation was applied to different nerves? The same sensation, it was learnt, as would happen by mechanical or chemical irritation, and as occurred naturally. Electrical reactions could therefore be used for examining the functions of the nervous system. Electrical stimulation applied to nerves gave a better understanding of how the voluntary and involuntary muscles contracted; those, as in the arms and the legs, under direct, conscious control; and those, as in the blood vessels, stomach, heart, lungs and internal organs, not under direct conscious control.

Another important step in discerning the functions of the nervous system was the analysis of "reflex actions", the puzzle of the involuntary sneeze. It was learned that where there was an immediate response to a stimulation, "messages" passed directly through the spinal cord without being first sent to the brain; a simple illustration was the jerking of the limbs which could be induced in a frog by chemical or electrical irritation of the skin, even after the brain had been destroyed. This interesting phenomenon also cast more light on actions such as standing, breathing and walking, which generally appear to be maintained at a level just below consciousness. As a result of these and further studies, it became clear that the brain and the nervous system played an important part in preserving the harmony and health of the internal environment of the body in its reaction with the changing external environment.

While this important work continued, other schools of medical thought were concentrating on the functions of the individual organs of the body, gaining a knowledge of their structure in general and in detail, and studying various deviations from normal. With an increase in post-mortem studies, it was possible to group together various symptoms and associate them with specific organs; a discerning pathologist, however, stated in criticism: "It is not the dead organ that medicine wishes to understand, but the living organ, exercising the functions peculiar to it." Nevertheless, important advances were made on these lines, particularly in hospitals well equipped with pathological departments.

This was a time of great successes in the age-long search for specific diseases. At the great London hospital of Guy's, brilliant team-work under the leadership of outstanding doctors resulted in a number of famous discoveries, including Bright's disease of the kidneys, Addison's disease of the adrenal glands, and Hodgkin's disease of the lymphatic glands. Ireland also distinguished itself with a group of clinicians in Dublin whose names will always be associated with pioneer medical research: Graves, Corrigan, Stokes and Cheyne. Two thousand years before, Hippocrates had watched with helpless sympathy the laboured breathing of a dying patient; Cheyne and Stokes made the same observation and were able, through modern knowledge of the circulation, to relate it to a disturbance in the action of the heart.

Practising doctors began to rely more on the laboratory; and with the development of more efficient instruments to aid observation and measurement, the clinicians were encouraged still more to concentrate on the study of individual organs. So much so, that it was succinctly observed of nineteenth-century medicine: "The road to the clinic goes through the pathological museum."

The Tools for the Job

Medical equipment was added to by one splendid improvement and invention after another.

A boyish game of listening through hollow logs to the resonant sound of tapping inspired the invention of the stethoscope; and the thermometer, which had been invented 100 years before, was improved and applied to studying the heat of the body in disease. The blood-pressure apparatus was introduced first in France, and was of great value in the study of heart and blood-vessel disorders.

Then the most amazing of all modern inventions began to be applied to medical use. Electricity, which had brought light to the darkest places, was now harnessed to instruments which the doctor could turn on the inner recesses of the body. With the ophthalmoscope he could view the retina of the eye; the laryngoscope lit up the dark passage of the throat; and with the cystoscope the bladder could be clearly seen. How much obscurity was dispelled by these beautiful instruments! Even more sensitive were the machines for recording the electrical impulses of the heart, which reached their greatest refinement with the production of the electro-cardiograph.

All the factors of ill health that could be weighed, measured or chemically analysed, were submitted to these new methods of investigation. The experimental pathologist began to abstract the chemicals contained in the blood and in the diseased organs, and the discovery of these substances gave important clues to the nature of the trouble.

The doctor at the bedside was now able to receive more scientific help, and no longer had to rely on intuition and guesswork as his only guides. He also began to pay less attention to the symptoms which were described by the patient, and which are not easily gauged, and looked more closely at the signs which could be studied with scientific detachment, with the help of all the fine new machines. The centre of this school of medicine was Vienna, which gained and retained a high reputation for brilliant diagnosis of disease; but the sick man as a whole was often forgotten in the meticulous investigations into his diseased organs.

The microscope had already revealed to a handful of scientists vitally important secrets of nature; and in this age of machines, its structure was soon improved until it was able to give a perfectly clear and unclouded view to a very high degree of magnification. The all-important tissues were submitted to its searching light; and then there emerged a fascinating new theory of medicine centred round the cells, which were seen as the basic units of tissues.

The Cell—Lowest Common Factor of Life

All living tissue, from a starfish to a star-gazer, could be reduced to the lowest common factor: the microscopic cell, one of a colony of millions and billions, each with its nucleus. The cells were individual units, with a life of their own, yet they were also an integral part of the larger organism which they constituted. What was more, plants, animals and men all arose from a single cell which contained within itself the power to multiply until it had fulfilled its own particular destiny. Aristotle had initiated the science of embryology when he traced the progress of the unborn chick within the egg. This new knowledge of the cell retold the beginning of the story and also helped towards completing it.

The discovery of cells by German scientists soon led biologists into discussions and experiments of the greatest significance. It appeared that cells had a variety of adventures when disease struck at the body. In apparently unaffected organs, some cells degenerated and died, while in severely damaged organs, numbers of cells remained unharmed in a battlefield strewn with the dead and dying. The various changes in the cells and organs in inflammation and in different fevers helped in distinguishing many conditions which until then had all been considered as a single disease.

Doctors were encouraged to specialise. "Let us concentrate on the affected part, and we shall be able to control the disease", they argued.

Virchow led the famous Viennese School of Medicine in the new theory of the cell. He saw the body as "a cell-state" in which "every cell is a citizen" and disease "merely a conflict of citizens in this state brought about by the action of external forces".

There was no room in this theory for the Darwinian story of life struggling with the environment, and changing and evolving new forms in the process; neither could much credit be given to the theory of disease arousing the body to increase its defensive chemical mechanism to overcome the invading germs.

Here was the basis for a dispute of international proportions. From all the European universities the giants of the profession entered the debate, expostulating with and contradicting each other; but after the heat of argument had cooled, they returned to their laboratories and began to search with renewed zeal for the elusive truth.

Virchow's insistence on the part played by cells in disease was reinforced by Metchnikoff, who showed that white blood corpuscles flowed in the blood vessels, ever on the alert for invading germs or foreign bodies, which they could pounce upon and destroy. Naturally, followers of the school of chemical changes and of antitoxins in the body could not accept the cell theory entirely.

Both schools had discovered some aspect of the truth, but as they had failed to reconcile their knowledge, both tended to arrive at false conclusions.

The most important contribution made by Virchow was the understanding he gave doctors regarding new growths, particularly cancer. It was clear from his studies that growths resulted from specific cells multiplying rapidly and spreading at the expense of other cells in the body.

What of the Patient?

The stirring controversies, experiments and triumphs of the scientific world brought about some changes in medical practice. As far as the ordinary man was concerned, an occasional sensational head-line or garbled rumour about a life-saving discovery led to a momentary hope that the miraculous cure, so long sought after, had at last been found; but the moment passed, and people would return once more to the ancient medical myths, re-named according to modern fashions.

While the more progressive doctors were basing treatment on the latest work of the chemists and physiologists, many others were prac-tising as though they were still in the pre-scientific days, prescribing large helpings of a variety of drugs, irrespective of their action; and even blood-letting had its devotees. In fact, Professor Broussais, a surgeon in the French Army, was instrumental in raising the num-bers of leeches imported into France, and hundreds were used daily on his orders. And this high priest of the blood-letting ritual was honoured by the name of "The Messiah of Medicine".

The growing industry of Germany at this time led to the building of many laboratories, and medical knowledge made great headway in that country and in Austria. More attention, however, was paid to the mechanics of diagnosis and examination, than to the humane and psychological aspects of treatment; there was a danger of the disease becoming the centre of interest, to the exclusion of the patient for whose sake, presumably, the whole elaborate structure of scientific research had been established.

Since primitive times, the use of herbs and drugs had been an important part of the practitioner's equipment; the great sum of knowledge had been built up entirely by trial and error, but now it was the turn of these ancient prescriptions to come under the search-light of science. Drugs were analysed to separate out their chemical constituents, and these were examined to discover the effects they produced. Work commenced with that early example of man's ill-directed ingenuity—the poisoned arrow-head. Thousands of years ago men had known that curare introduced into the wound would hasten the kill; now it was possible to find out the reason.

Experiments showed that drugs acted specifically on certain organs and tissues; and this suggested a most important new line in the art of healing, for if drugs could affect healthy organs adversely, surely it would be possible to reverse the process?

Tests proved that a number of drugs were really useless for the purpose for which they had been taken, and better alternatives were found; another step forward led pharmacologists to isolate the active principal in the herb. Morphia was abstracted from opium in the beginning of the nineteenth century; and within the next few years, other essential aids to treatment were refined from their original source, as quinine from cinchona, strychnine from nux vomica, caffeine from coffee, and the pain-killer cocaine from a South American plant.

Nor was this all. Many of the substances found in nature which had curative qualities, could now be made artificially with chemicals in the laboratory, and a whole industry of synthetic drug-making was born. Some of the drugs could not be digested in the stomach, but that difficulty was soon overcome by the introduction of the hypodermic needle; once more a mechanical aid had been enlisted in the battle for health.

There was every incentive to continued experimenting in the laboratory with the action of chemicals; there seemed no limit to the cures that were waiting to be found. There was also the unpleasant discovery that certain drugs which had customarily been prescribed together were contradictory and harmful in their joint action; no one could tell how many patients had suffered as a result of this ignorance. One sad instance is that of Robert Burns whose last illness was certainly complicated by the simultaneous administration of both laudanum and mercury.

Other discoveries, however, were more positive. Apart from the useful application of amyl nitrite, digitalis and other heart stimulants, the blessing of effective anaesthesia was made possible by the use of cocaine as a local and spinal anaesthetic at the end of the nineteenth century, when there appeared also that universal panacea for all aches and pains, the household drug, aspirin.

Similar investigations into the effect of poisons and methods of counteracting them led to improvements in many dangerous industrial occupations, and in the detection of crime.

What other benefits could the more enlightened doctors confer upon their hopeful patients? Looking backward and passing over the chaos of the Middle Ages, they recalled the splendid hygiene of the classical world of Greece and Rome. Special baths, massage and physical culture were again applied after a searching investigation similar to those given to other forms of treatment. The chemical character of mineral springs was studied, and throughout Europe, Spas favoured by nature became established as the special preserve of wealthy patients of highly-placed practitioners.

At the end of the nineteenth century, the first Chair of Hydrotherapy was established at Vienna; and the first Professor, William Winternitz, carried out his duties with typical thoroughness. It is related of him that in one of his experiments he gave himself "a wet pack" in an extremely cold basement, and had to be dug out of the block of ice in which he was embedded as the water froze. Cold douches and cold draughts of water were introduced for treating fever, and in contrast the soothing power of heat was applied to affected parts. These forms of treatment, however, were not studied as intensively as were drugs and chemicals; and they tended to be vulgarised and exploited by unqualified practitioners.

The general practitioner began to suit his dress to the rational character of his profession. Gone at last were the trappings and trimmings of a magic craft; instead of fear and awe, the austere figure of the typical Victorian doctor inspired his patients with quiet confidence. The doctor gained support from the new sciences of bacteriology and cellular pathology. He could forget the impressive but meaningless Latin phrases; he was talking now in terms of a more exact science; at least so it seemed by comparison with the dim but not so distant past. Medicine had now its own professional journals. In Britain at the beginning of the nineteenth century, *The Lancet* and the *British Medical Journal* appeared.

Of all the sciences, medicine came most intimately into contact with people—with humanity engaged in the elemental struggle to avoid sickness. The young science of medicine had to function in a very complex world where there was nothing of the calculated order

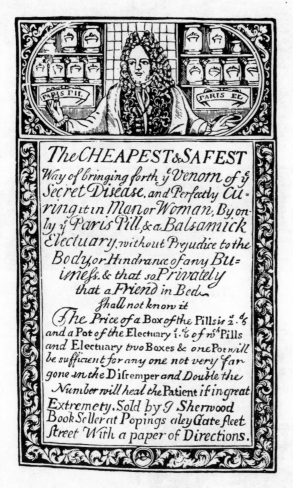

Advertisement.

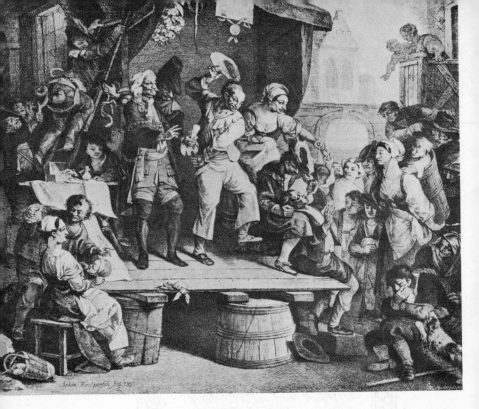

Travelling quacks.

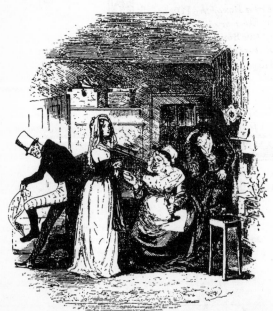

Sairy Gamp, the disreputable nurse in *Martin Chuzzlewit* by Charles Dickens.

of a laboratory. It was a test not only of medicine, but also of the medical practitioner.

Medicine for the Masses

Progress as a result of the new knowledge seemed to take place at different rates throughout the community. At the top level, great advances had been made, and some immediate benefits were being reaped by a small section of society—those who could afford to engage the well-informed medical man. For the great majority, illness was a disaster which could lead them only into the hands of quacks and charlatans, and finally through the narrow doors of the few dispensaries and infirmaries which grudgingly received them for free treatment.

People knew well enough that tremendous discoveries had been made which had moved even the scientists to astonishment and sudden optimism. Even to the ignorant the optimism was contagious, and every catchpenny charlatan was able to cash in on a vast market which could not afford the genuine article.

The development of the popular press helped greatly in this campaign. People suffering from various types of ailments were only too ready to believe the printed word, even if it was obviously an advertisement and the advertiser someone with a vested interest. Patent medicines were announced which claimed to cure anything from constipation to an unwanted pregnancy. Every journal from daily newspapers to religious magazines carried countless advertisements.

This form of pill-peddling became more widespread as people lost confidence in the possibility of obtaining practical help from medical scientists. The new advances had remained remote from the people; they had brought about the end of the charm-and-amulet school of mystical medicine, but no universal panacea had emerged as a result of the scientists' labours. Other sciences had produced practical and useful benefits, railways, telephones and the telegraph; what had medical research produced which could capture the public imagination and enthusiasm? The important sanitary reforms resulting from better medical knowledge made little appeal to those suffering from personal discomfort, and not accustomed to considering themselves as part of a highly organised social unit.

But the public yearned for some universal cure-all because the vast majority were sunk in an unhealthy environment, during both work and leisure.

In this favourable atmosphere, the masters of mass psychology stepped in to make fortunes for themselves, and fools out of a gullible public. A typical example was the career of the self-styled "Professor" Thomas Holloway, who smothered almost everybody with the widespread application of Holloway's Family Ointment, advertising in newspapers (literally) from China to Peru. The Great Pyramid itself served as a poster-site for an advertisement of his Universal Pill. He left hundreds of thousands of pounds; paradoxically, much of this fortune went in endowments for genuine medical establishments. Holloway's sardonic motto was the line from Dante, "And time shall see thee cured of every ill".

Holloway was no freak salesman; there were at least five millionaires living in London at the same period whose wealth had been made out of patent medicines. Purgative pills and soothing syrups were the most lucrative lines, and so vicious was the prescription for the innocuous-seeming syrup that at least 15,000 children each year were reckoned to have died in England as a result of the drug. Nearly a ton of laudanum was used in a year by one apothecary in producing the popular form of "baby-soother" which was given to children to keep them quiet while mothers were working. At best some of these "remedies" were ineffective and harmless, but many were positively harmful.

The European working population were receiving treatment for their aches and pains at the hands of ill-trained quacks, and paying heavily for the privilege. There was not always a clear dividing line between the regular medical practitioners who had "systems" for curing all ailments, or who recommended purgings or bleedings without restraint, and the unorthodox practitioners with *their* "systems", usually much more entertaining.

This was the era of the greatest showman of them all, Barnum, whose happy hunting ground was among the polyglot immigrants to the New World; other showmen with a sound business sense developed the "health for all" theme, which paid such excellent dividends. In New York alone, during the eighteen-forties, over 100,000 dollars a year were spent on advertising various "secret" cure-alls.

All types of health sects flourished; the vegetarians, the wholemeal adherents and other food faddists, the herbalists, the believers in "water-treatment", and the modern version of the Greek Temple healers, the Christian Scientists. These different sects had their prophets and their followers, and no doubt their silent martyrs. They were also well-established in the commercial field, and over eighty journals dedicated to different health-reform movements were published in the United States alone between 1830 and 1890.

The Profession puts its House in Order

This unseemly scramble to make quick money out of medicine had to be curbed. The Profession fitted into the general run of affairs and required a profitable return for services rendered, but it was felt that it should at least conduct itself with dignity.

High-sounding colleges of medicine soon appeared on both sides of the Atlantic, but often their most important activity was collecting fees. For one winter's attendance at lectures, colleges would accommodate the student with a diploma certifying him as a full-fledged doctor.

In Great Britain an effort was made at the beginning of the nineteenth century to standardise at least the minimum requirements of technical education, and it was laid down by Act of Parliament that the practitioners could make a charge only for drugs. The main effect of this was to lengthen the size and number of prescriptions.

A variety of colleges turned out a stream of more or less qualified people, including bone-setters and herbalists; and so the patient had a bewildering choice of charlatans, all of them claiming the status of doctor or surgeon. Many medical bodies emerged from the religious and trade guilds of the Middle Ages, but their long tradition was no guarantee of their integrity in granting licences.

An effort was made to co-ordinate the education and organisation of the medical profession. At the beginning of the nineteenth century, the Royal College of Surgeons was founded, and to counter the multiplication of teaching "colleges", medical training was begun in the hospitals. Several thousand private doctors were appointed officially to give some of their time to the treatment of the poor; and within fifty years, Britain had public vaccinators, and part-time medical officers of health. An official Medical Council was set up to regulate the activities of about 20,000 doctors, a number which bears a similar proportion to the population of today. Unsuitable practitioners could be removed from the register; but the standards were low, and there was a continuous struggle to protect the public from deception and to maintain the good name of the Profession.

From Sairy Gamp to Florence Nightingale

From earliest history it has been the woman's part to comfort the weak, but in most times society extended little encouragement or respect to those who exercised this function to succour the sick and diseased. From the Middle Ages onwards, nursing was so ill-paid and thankless a task that it degraded the best, and generally attracted only the worst of ignorant and hardened characters. Who else could stand the strain of those overcrowded, unsavoury hospitals, of having usually to care for nearly twenty ill people at a time, or of acting as night-nurse to at least 100 helpless and hopeless patients; the yearly salary for this drudgery was usually no more than a domestic worker could earn: about five pounds.

However, in case even these conditions might prove too attractive to patients by comparison with home comforts, the Poor Law Commissioners recommended that medical relief of the poor should not be encouraged to reach too high a standard. In the middle of the nineteenth century, the 600 workhouses and poor law infirmaries maintained by State benevolence averaged only one paid nurse for every two establishments, so there was hardly any of the danger feared by the Mr Bumbles of the Poor Law Commission.

People who were compelled to enter hospital because they had infectious diseases had an even worse reception. In the gloomy, cold and un-aired infectious disease hospitals they lay, often two to a bed, with no one but themselves to attend to them. They had to empty their bed-pans and slops, and recovery was more a question of good fortune than of medical skill. Many of those who were discharged left hospital with a new ailment, such as ringworm, or unwillingly sheltering that too-friendly companion, the louse.

Not all the sick requiring nursing could, or would, enter hospital.

For them there was always the service of the typical Victorian handy-woman-nurse, immortalised by Charles Dickens in the person of Sairy Gamp. Let the author describe her: "The face of Mrs Gamp —the nose in particular—was somewhat red and swollen, and it was difficult to enjoy her society without becoming conscious of a smell of spirits. Like most persons who have attained to great eminence in their profession, she took to hers very kindly; . . . she went to a lying-in or a laying-out with equal zest and relish." And always dressed in the same "rusty black gown, rather the worse for wear"; she could not think of visiting a case without the shawl, the bonnet, and the germ-laden old umbrella. Sairy Gamp, naturally, had to have some means of increasing her uncertain income, and she had a ladylike arrangement with Mr Mould, the prosperous undertaker, whereby, for a small commission, she would readily recommend potential customers.

It is impossible to part from Sairy without giving a description of at least one of the many scenes which reveal the state of private nursing of those not too distant times. Here she is, calmly eating her supper while the old man who is her patient is showing serious signs of some nervous disturbance.

" 'Why, highty tighty, sir !' cried Mrs Gamp, 'is these your manners? You want a pitcher of cold water throw'd over you to bring you round; that's my belief.' When she had finished the last crumb, Mrs Gamp took him by the collar of his coat, and gave him some dozen or two of hearty shakes backward and forward in his chair; that exercise being considered by the disciples of the Prig school of nursing (who are very numerous among professional ladies) as exceedingly conducive to repose, and highly beneficial to the performance of the nervous functions. Its effect in this instance was to render the patient so giddy and addle-headed, that he could say nothing more; which Mrs Gamp regarded as the triumph of her art."

The population was increasing rapidly in all the highly industrialised countries, and sooner or later adequate hospitals and decent nursing had to be provided. In the first quarter of the nineteenth century, Great Britain had built no fewer than 154 hospitals, and a capital city like Paris was able to accommodate 20,000 patients. Hospitals were equipped with X-ray, anaesthetic and other expensive equipment, and the patient was at last as well served as the animal in a laboratory experiment. These scientific machines called for skilled and qualified people to handle them, and the era of the de-humanised pauper's nurse drew to a close.

The end came with the beginning of a drive for higher standards of nursing, led and inspired by the magnificent work of Florence Nightingale. The most important outcome of the Crimean War was the fight she waged in the crowded army hospital at Scutari. She created a revolution in treating sick and wounded soldiers. Her struggle was not only against disease, but also against bureaucracy, inefficiency and the traditionally callous attitude of authority towards people needing medical care.

The work Florence Nightingale began under emergency conditions was continued in peacetime; and she helped to establish a school and home for nurses in St Thomas's Hospital, where it was at last recognised that the goodwill towards sick people which turns most people towards nursing, must be encouraged and trained in a scientific way. Religious training was no longer considered essential, but good character was insisted upon; and thousands of women began to take up a career which had been raised from the level of domestic work to the status of a profession.

The enthusiastic disciples of Florence Nightingale campaigned with her for those things which were essential to effective nursing: light, warmth, well-cooked and well-served meals, and above all, cleanliness.

Their successful efforts were probably the most positive contribution of the nineteenth century to the health of the community, although in other directions great strides were being made to help adjust the balance between the inward and outward environment so essential to man's well-being.

Chapter Eight

THE INDUSTRIAL REVOLUTION (2)

THE world-shaking impact of the Industrial Revolution had telescoped centuries of history into a few decades. Men had lived to see the creation of more wonders in a generation than had been produced in a millennium: steam-power, electricity, telegraphy, the X-ray, the microscope and many others. Man had learnt the secrets of his own body, of the existence of the cell, of the story of evolution; surely with all this knowledge humanity was on the threshhold of a truly civilised existence? Had not man forged for himself the means of mastering his environment? The scientific achievements and the industrial output of the century made such aims seem possible; but how, in cold reality, were these potential masters of the universe living?

Go back from today only 100 years or so, to the England of the early nineteenth century, the foremost industrial country in the world, the land of greatest promise. In a quaint little hamlet in the county of Cheshire, an agricultural worker looks hopelessly at his hungry and ragged family; in this neglected and almost deserted backwater, there is little hope of keeping his family alive on the few shillings he can earn from farming; in fact, he can scarcely pay for the scrap of bacon rind that occasionally flavours the bowl of broth or leeks that is his daily, unchanging diet. It would be no hardship to leave the dismal cottage with the leaky roof; the cottage without light, air or water, where the whole family are crowded into one room in an atmosphere heavy with all the despair of poverty and frustration. But what can they do? A member of the family who has received the blessing of civilisation and can read, discovers a message of salvation in a local paper. He sees an announcement, as do thousands of other dispossessed and unwanted land-workers: "To families desirous of settling in Macclesfield, wanted 4,000 to 5,000 people between the ages of seven and twenty-one."

Salvation indeed. Not only to some members of the Cheshire

family, and thousands like them, but to the streams of demobilised soldiers returning from the Napoleonic wars, to the emigrant Irish labourers driven from their own neglected countryside to seek a living far from home, and to the dwindling fraternity of craftsmen whose excellent skills could no longer earn them even the price of a loaf of bread.

Salvation, indeed. To the profit-hungry owners of mill and factory, out to sweep the world with a torrent of goods pouring in a never-ending flow from the costly machines. To reap the rich rewards, they must have hands, old and young, gnarled and tender; hands must keep the machines going night and day, day and night. But they had little to fear. Sheer necessity drove whole populations into the growing towns; Manchester and midland towns like Birmingham expanding ten-fold in the first fifty years of the century, and small but conveniently placed villages like Bradford and Oldham increasing 100 times.

The beating heart of the town was the ever-thumping machine; houses, warehouses and factories were built in hasty and haphazard confusion. There was no time, nor any thought for planning. Even with careful attention, it would have been difficult to cope with the problems of water supply, drainage, and adequate housing and ventilation needed to keep this vastly increasing population in good health. As it was, employers were concerned only with the healthy state of their banking accounts; and workers with the receipt of that weekly pay packet essential to their survival.

Before this driving storm the warning voices of the few far-sighted sanitary-reformers seemed like whispers in a whirlwind. The workers themselves were unable to see the consequences of the tremendous social upheaval in which they were taking part. The lessons were soon to be learnt in affliction and sorrow, with hundreds of thousands of people wiped out by contagious diseases.

In the meantime, the hard-pressed people packed their few belongings and flocked to the towns, for they had to live somehow. Once again, that fierce chronicler of the industrial revolution, Dickens, forces us to see the new conditions as clearly as if we, too, had been one of these migrant folk:

"It was a town of red brick, or of brick that would have been red if the smoke and ashes had allowed it; but, as matters stood, it was a town of unnatural red and black, like the painted face of a savage. It was a town of machinery and tall chimneys, out of which interminable serpents of smoke trailed themselves for ever and ever, and never got uncoiled. It had a black canal in it, and a river that ran purple with ill-smelling dye, and vast piles of building full of windows where there was a rattling and a trembling all day long, and where the piston of the steam engine worked monotonously up and down like the head of an elephant in a state of melancholy madness. It contained several large streets all very like one another, and many small streets still more like one another, inhabited by people equally like one another, who all went in and out at the same hours, with the same sound upon the same pavements, to do the same work, and to whom every day was the same as yesterday and tomorrow, and every year the counterpart of the last and next."

That could have been Birmingham, Newcastle, Sheffield, or the industrial quarters of London. In dreary and monotonous rows of houses, people lived without any comfort or convenience. They slept often five or six to a bed, which was usually no more than a heap of rags on the floor. In the mining villages the beds never grew cold, accommodating both day and night shifts of workers in turn.

The authorities responsible for the large towns showed no interest in supplying adequate lighting or water supplies to the poorer quarters, where most of the population lived. There was usually only one stand-pipe for supplying water to fifteen or twenty houses, and the disposal of sewage was so badly arranged that the unpleasant smell from the Thames frequently distracted the attention of Parliamentary Committees and even at one period forced the Law Courts to close.

Some courageous medical officers spoke out strongly in their reports, using such unofficial language as "infernal", and shocked phrases describing "one universal atmosphere of filth and stink" where the poor lived, "in damp, dirty, stinking holes", and in conditions which were "hotbeds of nuisance and disease".

The reaction of people of power and position was to remove themselves as far as possible from these unpleasant conditions. Landlords devoted their profits from the hideous slums to provide healthy accommodation for themselves on high ground on the outskirts of the town; where they made sure to obtain a good water supply and adequate drainage, as recommended by the best medical authorities.

Dr Southwood Smith put the matter in a nutshell in his report of 1838: "While systematic efforts on a large scale have been made to widen the streets, to remove obstruction to the circulation of free currents of air, to extend and perfect the drainage and sewerage, and to prevent the accumulation of putrefying animal and vegetable substances in the places in which the wealthier classes reside, nothing whatever has been done to improve the conditions of the districts inhabited by the poor."

"The Dark, Satanic Mills"

The evil effects of the dreadful home conditions which helped to undermine resistance and spread infectious diseases were greatly augmented by the slum factories where the workers spent nearly all their time.

The structure of factory organisation had been so impatiently improvised; who gave a thought to the comfort or welfare of the workers? In fact, any suggested interference by outside authorities would have been bitterly opposed by the new barons of Britain, the manufacturers and industrialists. They wholeheartedly upheld the doctrine of "laisser faire"; in other words, complete freedom for the business man to further his own interests in any way he wished. This sort of freedom was certainly bringing in the profits, but there was another side to the picture which was anything but profitable in terms of the well-being of the people, and certainly not a pretty picture to study.

"The dark satanic mills" which now disfigured England's green and pleasant land were no fevered nightmare of the poet; in these gaunt buildings England's children were put to work from the age of three and four years; wages were so low that every member of the family must labour twelve hours a day and more to earn enough to pay the landlord and the baker. If the children so far forgot themselves as to drop exhausted by the machines to which they were bound (often literally, with chains), there was the overseer (recalling ancient, doomed Egypt), ready to beat them.

Parents had some choice of careers for their children. There was the mine, which welcomed the conveniently small stature of the five- and six-year olds; and for the more agile there was always a good opening in the chimney-sweeping trade. The mill and the factory, however, claimed the essential labour power of the great majority of "hands", and in these places the people spent the major part of their lives.

What were they like, these palaces of the kings of industry? In general, dirtier and gloomier than prisons, and smellier than refuse dumps; windows that were not tight-shut were blocked in to avoid the infamous window-tax. In a damp and often hot atmosphere, men, women and children toiled from five in the morning to nine at night; when business was good they worked longer hours, from three a.m. to ten p.m., and night work simply meant working continuously, the worker snatching a little sleep by the side of the machine, with no chance of seeing the sun or breathing fresh air for stretches of forty-eight hours or more.

If all this seems far removed from our modern ideas of common humanity, let it be recalled that there are people alive today whose grandparents accepted it as part of the established scheme of things. As late as 1842, a Law had to be passed in Parliament forbidding women, and children under ten years old, to work underground in the mines. Needless to say, even when a Law is passed, ways and means are found of avoiding it; and time must pass before it is fully respected.

These new ways by which people earned their bread began to produce a number of medical conditions, classified under a broad heading, "occupational diseases"; hospitals and surgeries often received patients suffering from such effects of their work as lead poisoning, silicosis, grinders' rot, potters' asthma, phosphorous ("phossy") jaw, mercurial poisoning and other unpleasant disorders. Accidents at work were common, and increased in number with the "speed-up" of the machines; in the mines they often took the form of large-scale disasters; yet children were frequently put in charge of the "safety" measures, leaving the experienced hands available for the "more important" work.

The workers who escaped serious injuries to health were nevertheless affected by the industries which employed them. They were not a handsome people, these children of the Industrial Revolution: pale, sickly, and stunted in growth through lack of suitable food and exercise in childhood, those who survived the gruelling test of the early years reached maturity with one minor disfigurement or other. Curvature of the spine, flat feet and bad posture were common, and ailments like varicose veins, digestive troubles and bronchitis seemed as inevitable as the autumn rains.

The Staff of Life

Man cannot live by bread alone, but he certainly cannot live without it. Since the shrewd businessman was always keen to supply a demand, he very soon turned his attention to developing a highly profitable source of sales: the food of the people.

There had been a time, not so long before, when people had lived close to the earth and had in many ways been able to satisfy their basic needs by the toil of their own hands; at least, what they had eaten had been fresh and wholesome, if not choice or even abundant. Millions now had stony pavements between them and the soil, and the grim back-to-back houses had no green gardens or space enough for a chicken run. But eat they must, and so the merchants became busy, not of course to help the workers to maintain a healthy and well-balanced diet—what had that to do with business?—but to pursue a new and promising avenue for free enterprise.

Free from any of the restraints that exist today, with only the beginning of public health and food inspection regulations, the men with capital went into the manufacture and sale of foodstuffs in an organised business-like way.

Always ready to use science in their own interests, many food manufacturers employed skilled chemists to dress up inferior foods to appear better and more costly than they really were. Chicory was sold as coffee, margarine (without the vitamins) as butter, cotton oil or mineral oil as olive oil. Milk was often watered, and had colouring matter added to make it appear creamy. Even worse, from the health aspect, was the way milk was produced, under the most filthy conditions and often from diseased cows; if that was not enough to make it really poisonous, it was stored in dirty cellars and hawked through the streets in open, unwashed containers, with polluted water added.

As is still common, the cheapest foods were least worth the hard-earned money that had to be paid. Potatoes and vegetables were frequently old and stale, bacon rancid, and meat the toughest and worst cuts, and usually beginning to go "off". Bread frequently had unwitting additions to its proper constituents: dead cockroaches, cobwebs and other unpleasant extras gathered from the bake-house; alum, sand, and other mineral substances were added by order of the "boss".

To make quite sure of their customers, many industries had their own company-store where workers were compelled to buy, with a debit calculated against their wages. These canny employers thus forged another weapon to slash the value of the wages they had to pay.

Consequently, tuberculosis was the disease that found most victims among a population undernourished, over-worked and overcrowded by day and night. It was so common that it became a familiar theme of the Victorian novelist who wished to wring an easy tear from the reader. The delicate, fading heroine had only to have the suggestion of "consumption" to make her interesting. However, the stories rarely dealt with the grim reality which turned the pleasantly sad fiction into unromantic human tragedy.

In these conditions, all the infectious diseases which had plagued the people of past eras flared up into typical old-fashioned epidemics, despite the advancing scientific knowledge of the day. From cholera and diphtheria right through the medical alphabet to typhoid and typhus, wherever people were herded together in factories, homes, mines and workhouses, the germs spread, striking in every direction. An unfamiliar enemy, Asiatic cholera, attacked the main European cities with all the ferocity of the plague. More than 50,000 people lost their lives in one attack; and in Paris, in the year 1831, during the height of an epidemic, thousands lay dead, and streams of refugees numbering 100,000 fled from the city.

The effect of a cholera epidemic in England was described in an official report to the Registrar-General in 1849, which read: "If a Foreign Army had landed on the coast of England, seized all the seaports, sent detachments over the surrounding districts, ravaged the population through the summer, after harvest destroyed more than a thousand lives a day for several days in succession, and in the year it held possession of the country, slain 53,293 men, women and children, the task of registering the dead would be inexpressibly painful; and the pain is not greatly diminished by the circumstance that in the calamity described the minister of destruction was a pestilence that spread over the face of the land and found in many cities quick poisonous matters ready at hand to destroy the inhabitants."

It was inevitable that infectious diseases should be rampant. In the ten years 1860-70 the London Fever Hospital alone dealt with 14,000 cases of typhus; not surprising when one recalls the official description of the homes of the poor as "damp, dirty, stinking holes". Dirt, lice and typhus were the three unholy links in the chain of disaster, and it was not much good trying to deal with the disease alone.

Other diseases like typhoid and cholera were spread by contaminated water, or through the innocent pale face of the milk which, beneath its creamy surface, hid dangerous germs, including those of scarlet fever and diphtheria. Scarlet fever killed one in every 500 children under the age of fifteen years, and diphtheria destroyed one in every thousand.

Even where the methods of protection had been known for some time, as in the case of vaccination for smallpox, they were not taken up by the Government as an essential form of prevention; the money that was grudgingly paid out went mainly to untrained and unskilled public vaccinators, so that smallpox was allowed to claim 400 out of each million of the population, in the years between 1871 and 1875. The melancholy records of 1871 tell also of the deaths of 70,000 people from the all-conquering tuberculosis germ, the king of destroyers.

This British tale of woe was repeated in the other advancing industrial countries, and although it received small mention in the history books, yet some of the events connected with these terrible epidemics had historical significance; for example, the very serious outbreak of yellow fever which hit Philadelphia, U.S.A., in 1783. The entire Federal Government threw dignity (and the security of the population) to the winds, and fled from the city. When the excitement had passed over, there was such a united drive for sanitary reforms that the city was given a water supply pumped by steam at the public expense; and so Philadelphia (the "city of brotherly love"), set the example for the whole of the English-speaking world.

Public Indignation and Public Conscience

The nineteenth century was not going blindly to repeat the experiences of the Middle Ages. People understood that they were living in an age of science, an age of power and promise. The advanced countries of the world were building up a modern civilisation of steel and concrete, yet millions were living far below the standards of human decency, their resistance to disease no stronger than it had been through the long dark centuries.

The people felt this paradox; and as poverty and sickness broke up and destroyed family after family, the "hungry" 'forties took on a deeper meaning and became the "angry" 'forties. The politicians were well aware of this rising indignation among the people; and on February 4, 1840, during a debate on social conditions in the House of Commons, it was moved that a committee be set up "to inquire into the causes of discontent among great bodies of the working-classes in populous districts". The reason given for this discontent was revealing: "the want of legislative provisions for the preservation of their health and the comfort of their homes."

The anger of the people at first led them to fruitless and savage attacks against the apparent cause of their torment, the machines; but though they broke their hands and their hearts against these heedless giants, their spirit was not broken; from the chaos and poverty, the working people organised themselves and there arose the magnificent movement of the British Chartists, with a demand for equal political rights for all people. It was not a question of a struggle for prestige or social position; the whole essence of Chartism was summed up in the phrase: "Political power our means, social happiness our end." The Chartist Petition which demanded higher wages and shorter working hours was soon signed by no less than three and a half million people; that is, by more than half the adult male population.

Public protest against intolerable injustice found a practical expression in the co-operative movement, which was created as a counter to the excessive greed of the mill-owners who used their monopoly of flour to keep up its price. The handful of working people who put their few shillings together and opened the first small "co-operative" shop in Rochdale in 1844, faced every obstacle, from the derision of many of the public to the deliberate hostility of established shop-keepers and wholesalers. However, the first co-operators had hungry families whose needs they were determined to satisfy, and the Rochdale pioneers succeeded in founding a movement which became world-wide.

Alongside the struggles of the working people, the public con-science found expression in the writings and work of many out-standing social reformers, novelists, lawyers, and above all, doctors whose whole training had taught them to dedicate themselves to the preservation of human life and well-being.

Charles Dickens and Emile Zola put into novel after novel their indignation at the degradation of human dignity which resulted from the poor and squalid lives most people were forced to lead. Robert Burns spoke for all his fellows whose deep poverty he had shared: "Man's inhumanity to man makes countless thousands mourn."

But for those of the strongest character, mourning was not enough. The foremost doctors and scientists found they could not keep their knowledge and understanding behind the closed doors of the study. Virchow, who was famed for his formulation of the cell-theory, declared boldly: "Medicine is a social science and politics nothing but medicine on a grand scale." He also wrote, "Doctors are the natural advocates of the poor, and social problems are largely within their jurisdiction"; and being an honest man, he practised what he preached. He investigated the troubles of the mill-workers of Silesia, and strongly condemned in the Prussian Reichstag the insanitary con-ditions he had seen. He advocated setting up a National Health Council, and was a bitter opponent of Bismarck. His activities natur-ally put him out of favour with the authorities, but the value of his work remained although they treated him with contempt.

Dr Southwood Smith, an eminent member of the British Board of Health, also believed that insofar as poverty affected the health of the people, it was for both the people and the Government to deal with it; but after meeting with indifference from the highest authorities, he turned to the real sufferers, the people, and in 1847 addressed them in a manifesto which said:

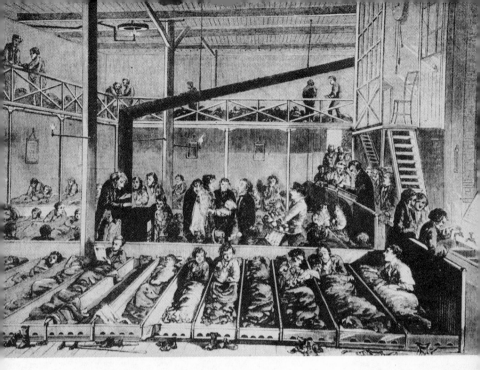

The Field Lane Refuge "for the destitute and homeless poor".

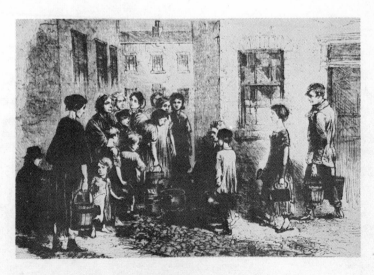

Single-tap water supply for houses in Bethnal Green.

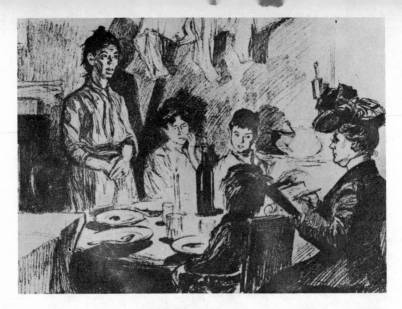

Health visitor.

A Potteries landscape.

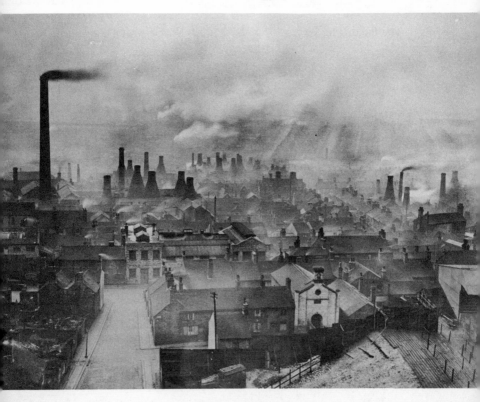

"For every one of the lives of these 1,500 persons who have perished during the last quarter and who might have been saved by human agency, those are responsible whose proper office is to interfere and to stay the calamity—who have the power to save but will not use it. But their apathy is an additional reason why you should rouse yourselves and show that you will submit to this dreadful state of things no longer. Let a voice come from your streets, alleys, courts, workshops and houses that shall startle the ear of the public, and command the attention of the Legislature."

People reading such a statement, even today, might consider it to come from some extremist political source, but it was in fact the sober opinion of a highly-placed official who saw that his first duty was the defence of health; and that duty he carried out with complete honesty.

In France, the struggle to bring practice into line with theoretical advances was championed by no less a figure than Pasteur. In one of his last speeches he made a memorable contribution to a debate that is still raging in our own times. He said:

"Two contrary laws seem to be wrestling with each other nowadays; the one, a law of blood and death, ever imagining new means of destruction and forcing nations to be constantly ready for the battlefield—the other, a law of peace, work and health, ever evolving new means of delivering man from the scourges which beset him.

"The one seeks violent conquests, the other the relief of humanity. The latter places one human life above any victory; while the former would sacrifice hundreds and thousands of lives to the ambition of one. The law of which we are the instrument seeks, even in the midst of carnage, to cure the sanguinary ills of the law of war; the treatment inspired by our antiseptic methods may preserve thousands of soldiers. Which of those two laws will ultimately prevail, God alone knows. But we may assert that French science will have tried, by obeying the law of Humanity, to extend the frontiers of Life."

The General Advance

The campaign for sanitary reforms at last won official recognition in the civilised world. Now it was down in black and white in every major language that the simple but essential laws of hygiene should be observed. Men had learned from the practice and experience of centuries, what was necessary: adequate water supplies, good drainage, supervision of lodging-houses, public baths, the clearing away of nuisances, the isolation of infectious disease.

But it was one thing to draw up regulations, another to see they were carried out. The highest authorities relied on the lower levels, the local administrators; and who were they? In the main, people of sufficient wealth and importance to achieve these positions. It was indeed unrealistic to expect owners of slum factories and slum properties to enforce improvements which they themselves would have to carry out. Despite the many new Acts that were passed, an authority like Dr Southwood Smith could protest that no sanitary improvements had been made in the working-class districts.

Yet, in sheer self-defence, people had to struggle on; supported by reformers like Chadwick and the Earl of Shaftesbury they compelled the Government to pass the various Factory Acts which at least formed the basis for protecting the interests of working women and children. Four inspectors were appointed to carry out the gigantic task of supervising thousands of factories up and down the country.

The New World of the United States repeated the European story, but in a cruder fashion. The Industrial Revolution had developed feverishly in this young and untried civilisation. Driven by chaotic forces, the populations re-created on virgin soil the old evils of the crowded cities of other lands. New York, as late as 1865, was described in a special survey as a place where "domestic garbage, filth and the refuse of the bedrooms of those sick with typhoid fever, scarlet fever and smallpox is frequently thrown into the streets, there to contaminate the air, and no doubt aid in the spread of these pestilential diseases". The survey established that 18,000 people at least were living in cellars, ". . . many below the high-water mark. At high tide the water often wells up through the floors, submerging them to a considerable depth. In very many cases, the vaults of privies are situated on the same or a higher level, and their contents frequently ooze through the walls into the occupied apartments beside them."

The ruthless elements in the community who had pushed their way to the top of the business world also took over the lucrative positions in local government, and under the thin cover of democratic forms, political corruption spread like contagious disease. In the face of a cholera epidemic in the early 'sixties, the Mayor of New York refused to call together the aldermen who constituted the Board of Health. He maintained, courageously, that these men were more dangerous to the City than the disease itself. He had some grounds for his words: a typical example was the item of one million dollars appropriated for the Street Cleaning Department: the filth remained in the streets, and the money went into hands which, in their own way, were equally dirty.

However, some action had to be taken when epidemics threatened to get beyond control; the knowledge was there, and the machinery could be set up and made to work for the general good, at least in an emergency. Every age finds the people who are able and willing to organise, and to sacrifice themselves, in the interests of the many. So in the 1840's, Southwood Smith formed "The Health of Towns Association" in England; and some years later in the United States, "Great American Congresses for Hygiene Reform" were held in Philadelphia, Baltimore and Boston.

As usual, progress was not made smoothly; but out of every conflict, the defenders of health emerged able to claim new victories.

Between 1860 and 1890, death from "fevers" was reduced by a half; the wider application of medical knowledge and improvements saved nine out of ten of those who would have died from smallpox in earlier days. Most notable was the victory over cholera, which disappeared from the United States in the 'seventies and from Western Europe by the end of the century. The tidal-waves of contagion were slowly, slowly being forced back; the balance of power was moving over to the side of man's conscious efforts against disease.

"All Hands on Deck"

An ambitious, steam-driven economy like that of Great Britain could no longer afford the disturbances caused by frequent epidemics. It was bad enough when machines broke down, but when they ceased working because the people who manned them were removed in great numbers by sudden fever and death, and when the farmlands lay untended and all the necessary business of private and public life came to a standstill, then it was time for a determined attack on the cause of these troubles.

Although there was not yet an exact knowledge of the way in which germs could affect water polluted by sewage, the accumulated experience of generations had produced awareness that infectious diseases were spread through dirty conditions. People naturally recoiled from bad smells and an unpleasant atmosphere, and it was almost universally held that these were the source of the trouble. So, for the wrong reasons, they began to do the right things at last.

The industrial manufacture of cast-iron pipes made it possible for pure water to be brought easily, economically, and uncontaminated on its long journey into the homes of the people. At last the noxious accumulation of civilised living could be taken away underground. Chemistry and physics were enlisted to make doubly sure of safety by treating the sewage to make it harmless, and purifying the water by methods of filtering.

Nevertheless, despite energetic drives against bad smells and "poisonous" vapours, epidemics still occurred. The experts were puzzled. Even Farr, who had carried out such important work in studying epidemics, concluded that it was healthier to live on high rather than low ground, but failed to see that it was safer there, not because the air was fresher, but because the houses were better constructed and had a purer water supply.

In 1854, a frightening epidemic of cholera broke out in the vicinity of Broad Street. Despite the efforts of many doctors, the epidemic continued in an unpredictable manner. The problem was finally solved by Dr John Snow, a physician to Queen Victoria. At a meeting of the authorities called to discuss the epidemic, he demanded the removal of the handle of the Broad Street pump. With much scepticism, his request was carried out. As he had predicted, there were no further cases of cholera, and there should have been no further doubt about the importance of pure water.

At that time, water was supplied as a commodity under schemes of free enterprise; investigations showed that the customers of one firm were dying at three and a half times the rate of those obtaining their supplies from a more hygienic source. The work of Snow and Farr had a salutary effect on all concerned, especially when further studies showed the relation of typhoid epidemics to contaminated water.

The medical profession was on the brink of discovering a momentous fact: the existence of disease-producing germs. In the ten years or so before Pasteur made the conclusive proof, certain far-sighted doctors were coming closer and closer in practice to the basic cause of many of their medical problems.

Cleanliness and good order were becoming more the general rule in hospitals; yet disasters still occurred which challenged the skill of the best doctors. For example, in maternity wards, the dreaded puerperal fever would strike mother after mother, and most of them would die in the face of all medical care. Two obstetricians, working independently, devoted all their thought to the defeat of this cruel killer. Oliver Wendell Holmes, an American, and Semmelweiss, a Hungarian, both came to the positive conclusion that whatever the cause of puerperal fever, it was spread by contagion, and the main precaution was scrupulous cleanliness in the ward and by the doctors handling the cases. They recommended using strong antiseptics, and clean clothes for the doctor on his rounds.

Then Semmelweiss shrewdly came close to the truth. He noted that a medical assistant died after an accidental wound which she sustained during a post-mortem on a mother dead from puerperal fever; the symptoms and the death were similar in both cases. He observed another significant fact: the death-rate in the hospital was greater when the students came straight from dissections in the post-mortem room to attend women in labour. His solution was simple; so simple that most doctors refused to admit what was indeed a devastating criticism of their own carelessness. "Wash your hands in antiseptic before examining the mothers," said Semmelweiss. This was something like Dr Snow's recommendation to remove the handle of the Broad Street pump; and it was disliked even more.

The contempt of his colleagues meant less to Semmelweiss than the lives of the women in his care. To his own students he insisted, "Wash your hands!" Within seven months the death-rate at his hospital was reduced to ten per thousand at a time when the average death-rate throughout the service was ten times higher.

Unhappily, mothers in every country continued to pay the price for the pride and prejudice of the profession in general. It took twenty years for them to accept the sense of Semmelweiss' teaching, and before that time their opposition and persecution drove him off his mental balance and he died insane.

There was nothing unusual in the treatment Semmelweiss received, although that was no comfort to him. Sir John Simon, the Chief Medical Officer of England, refused to accept the contamination theory of Dr Snow, and an exhibition of contempt was given by Max von Pettenkoffer, the famous German epidemiologist, who drank Dr Snow's health in a glass-full of cholera bacteria; fortunately for him he escaped the danger, but the correctness of Snow's surmise was proved conclusively by the experience of Pettenkoffer's fellow-countrymen in the year 1892. Water contaminated with cholera was supplied to Hamburg and Altona; Altona had a filtering system, and its population escaped infection; it was the citizens of Hamburg who suffered the horrors of a cholera epidemic.

The Culprit Nailed at Last

It had been a long and elusive chase. Leeuwenhoek had seen them first, the curious little dots and lines squirming under his home-made microscope. The most curious thing was that they were undoubtedly alive. Throughout the seventeenth century, other scientists peered through lenses, puzzling always how to find out more about these infinitesimal creatures. Slowly, they began to put together the life-story of bacteria, of which, even before Pasteur, the importance to plant and human life was recognised. Could it be that certain diseases were caused by the activities of unseen living things—parasites? Could they be friendly to man, helping him to digest his food, for example, as Spallanzani showed in the eighteenth century? What about that annoying disease that affected the silkworm? Even before Pasteur, the Italian Bassi was speculating about the possibility that it could—it *might* be the work of bacteria.

The search went on. In the middle of the nineteenth century Pasteur was devoting all his energy, skill and thought to this fascinating and tantalising study. All the past efforts of science seemed like a powerful force behind him, pushing him forward.

For the sake of their industry, the wine-merchants had backed

Pasteur generously during his research into the cause of fermentation. After exhaustive experiments, he proved without any doubt that micro-organisms could cause change, fermentation and disease. He applied his knowledge to a study of disease in silkworms, then sheep, and finally man. Pasteur's general laboratory work was not so well financed, but his labours proved of immeasurable benefit not merely to wine-merchants and silk dealers, but to mankind. He showed how germs invaded the living body and multiplied if the environment was favourable, so producing the ill-effects which had been only too well known to man.

Bacteriology was now the newest and most vital branch of medical science. Other bacteriologists were inspired by the wider possibilities of Pasteur's pioneering work. Koch, in Germany, set himself a formidable but tempting task: to detect the germ which caused each specific disease; he showed how to do this by isolating the germ, growing it outside the body, and with this same germ producing the disease in other animals and then isolating it again; thus enabling doctors to establish a complete mastery over the death-dealers, so that it would be possible to annihilate them.

The work in the laboratory went ahead steadily. Once again Pasteur was in the forefront in the new stage of the chase. Everyone was thinking along lines of strengthening the body's resistance to disease-germs; but how? Almost by accident, Pasteur discovered the method of inoculation which really did defeat the germs.

Returning from a much needed vacation, he picked up a specimen of chicken cholera virus which had been prepared for an experiment but had not been used; nevertheless, as part of the routine work, Pasteur injected the preparation into some chickens; the chickens, surprisingly, did not sicken and die, but the weakened germ stimulated their bodies to produce sufficient antitoxin so that they could overcome a further stronger injection of disease germs.

Like all the most profound discoveries, it seemed beautifully simple —once it was made. With the new knowledge, Pasteur was able to prepare an effective vaccine against anthrax which had previously killed millions of sheep and added to the poverty of the countryside; and in an atmosphere of great dramatic tension, he demonstrated the cure for hydrophobia on a number of Russian peasants who, after having been bitten by a mad wolf, had struggled half across Europe to be saved by the great Frenchman.

The work of Pasteur, Koch and their followers unmasked some of the worst marauders: typhoid, diphtheria, plague, cholera, tuberculosis, leprosy, syphilis. Small wonder that once again the rumour swept forward: the scientists were about to establish a final victory over disease. A long time before, it had been the charm, then the amulet; now the all-powerful theories of the cell and the germ, were to provide all the answers.

The germ theory was established, and made a complete change in the whole method and outlook of medicine. It gave the necessary extra stimulus to the authorities to provide a far better and more effective public health system, and it was being clearly demonstrated how the health and well-being of man was interwoven with the whole fabric of his environment.

The Way to Positive Health

Sanitary reforms could not stand still with merely defensive work against infection. If by keeping the cities free of dirt and the water supply uncontaminated, so many infant lives could be saved, what could not be achieved by positive action in promoting good health? The babies that in previous years would have been dead were now alive, in their mother's arms. The babies were a challenge and a stimulus. "You've kept us alive!" they seemed to say. "Now, what about preserving us from the lurking dangers?" Infant-care and management began to be a subject for the authorities as well as for parents so often ill-equipped to carry out unaided their important responsibilities. And if society was going to care in an organised way for the infant, what about the mother? If she could be saved from the tragedy of child-bed fever, it was only logical to extend care to the earlier period of pregnancy and help her to avoid the other complications which had so often brought death instead of new life. And so success in one direction led to hope and advance in many others.

With the encouragement of science and the conscious desire of the public, governments turned finally towards the road to social welfare. The protection of public health meant not only the control of disease, but also the control of the home environment and of un-healthy places of work, and the provision of personal health services in an ever-extending range. The people, too, were on the way to self-help, by forming societies and organisations which arranged finan-cial insurance against the hardship resulting from ill health. Germany set an example by taking government responsibility for social insur-ance. Although not all sections of society nor all governments were prepared to go the whole way, at least the course towards preventive and positive good health for the whole community was well and truly mapped out.

There was new hope for the community; the individual with his personal troubles could also face the doctor with a new confidence. The worst ordeal a sick or injured person had always endured was the knowledge that for the sake of the whole, some part of his body must be removed by medical intervention. Surgery had been the last resort of treatment up to the nineteenth century. Without knowledge of germ infection, it had indeed been a second-best to other forms of healing, and only an emergency or crisis had forced the decision.

Pain and shock alone could overcome the patient's powers of re-covery, although from the earliest days efforts had been made out of sheer pity to make the patient less conscious of his ordeal. Accord-ing to the custom and the period, opium, hemp, mandragora or a stiff drink of whisky had served a merciful function, and mesmerism or hypnosis had proved to different generations that it was possible to control the body through the mind. The certain control of anaes-thesia was finally achieved in the nineteenth century, with the dis-covery of ether and chloroform.

The surgeon was able at last to take his place as a life-saver beside the other powerfully-equipped men of medicine. The dreaded operating-theatre was now to be the scene of new and magnificent victories, its door opening to life and not to the mortuary.

The pioneer of the new antiseptic surgery was the English surgeon, Lister. Modern anaesthesia had made it possible to undertake longer and more complicated operations, but deaths through infection still occurred until the germ-theory was rigorously respected down to the smallest detail. Lister led the way by a determined use of the disinfectant spray in the wards and on the wounds of the patient.

Gradually, the inescapable truth that prevention was better than cure altered the methods of antisepsis.

A determined fight followed to exclude the germ from the entire radius of the operation with the help of surgical gowns, masks, rubber gloves, and in recent times, by filtering and purifying the air. How amazed old Galen would have been, with his theory of "laudable pus"; and how gratified those unnamed rebels of the thirteenth century, who preferred to follow Hippocrates and Celsus with their effort to keep wounds clean by washing with vinegar or wine.

With these two great advances, surgery now developed into a skill of the utmost delicacy and precision. The surgeon's knife dared to probe parts of the body no one had dreamed of operating on before: the nose, the ear, the eye, the throat, the abdomen, the chest, the brain—everything could be attempted, and greater successes followed on wider experience and improved technique. People no longer thought of themselves as "hopeless" surgical cases.

Mothers in particular gained from the new surgery. In the beginning of the nineteenth century, the ancient "Caesarean" operation to remove the living unborn child meant death for seven out of ten mothers. Antiseptic methods introduced with the new ideas took the terror out of this and other obstetric operations, and a growing understanding of the mechanism of labour encouraged an attitude of patient and watchful waiting rather than violent interference with a natural process.

What a hectic century medicine had passed through! From the horrors of children put to work at three years of age, to the glorious successes in reducing infant mortality by more than one-half through the work of a single generation of agitators, reformers and doctors.

The very pace of the industrial revolution had speeded up the actions and reactions of people. Just as poisons produced their antitoxins, so social evils worked on the social conscience and brought to life agitation and determination to see these things changed so that people could live their full span of life at the height of their powers.

The final test of the value of a mode of life is what happens to the children. In the middle of the eighteenth century three out of four children died before they reached the age of five years; by the beginning of the nineteenth century it had been reduced to two out of four. But the violent uprooting and re-directing of human beings with the coming of the industrial revolution had its inward strains exposed by the increase in infant mortality; the greatest triumph and the greatest justification of the struggle to better the condition of living was the protection of four out of five young lives from the strains of civilisation.

In fifty years the people had won a system of positive health protection, the development of infant and maternal care, clinics and school medical inspection. Doctors knew how to control the external environment which affected health, and they knew much of what was necessary to protect the individual from the worst effects of illness.

Clearly, health and happiness lay in the harmonious balance between man's inner and outer life. That perfect balance, however, was still far from having been attained.

Chapter Nine

THE TWENTIETH CENTURY

On the Shores of a New World

IT was the same old world, with the same old struggle to live and let live, the problem that had challenged man for hundreds and thousands of years. Yet it was a fantastically new world, changed in so short a period of fifty to 100 years, as it had not changed previously in dozens of generations. It was the twentieth century; the century of a new age, dazzling and terrible in its potentialities. The age of steel and concrete was being transformed into the atomic age, and at the centre man stood poised, moved by hopes and fears of awe-inspiring magnitude.

At first the way of progress had seemed so clearly and simply mapped out. All that was needed was time. In time, said the industrialists, we shall deal with the growing-pains of the new century. A few mild crises, some small slumps in trade causing sudden attacks of unemployment: these are undeniably painful while they last; but, is not the production of goods increasing? Every year we grow greater in our material possessions; and it seemed indeed that the markets of the world were insatiable. But what about the poverty of the producers, the people? Slums and preventable sickness are still with us, it was protested. Time, the leaders replied, all in good time.

The medical profession reflected this cheerful complacency. All in good time the new germ and cell theories would be applied to diseases which hindered men in their forward advance. Give us time, said the doctors, and we shall track down every germ and produce appropriate vaccines; we shall be able to protect people against every infection. There was similar optimism about the chances of remedying disorders of the organs of the body. Now that it was known that the body was made up of a variety of cells, all that was required was to study them and remedy any defects. It was a study the modern scientist appeared well-equipped to deal with. Once again, it seemed obvious that finding a cure for all afflictions was only a matter of time.

At the beginning of the century medical men already had some cause for confidence. After so many generations of doctors had relied mainly on inspired guesswork, modern practitioners could with reasonable accuracy discover what ailed the patient, and forecast the outcome. They could do so on the basis of the latest advance in medical knowledge, although with little aid from their instruments and testing apparatus, which by the standards of today can only be called crude. If they were not so successful in treatment, it was because the main source of ill-health was not yet determined, and the appropriate remedies were not always known. But at least the medical profession was becoming aware of its own ignorance and was prepared to learn from mistakes, generally from those revealed in the post-mortem room.

The Way Forward is Never in a Straight Line

The difficulties had been demonstrated over and over again; but the hope of an easy way seemed never to fade. Nevertheless, the century was not very old before disquieting experiences showed that both the world of science and the world of men were subject to complexities that would take some time to unravel. As far as the scientists were concerned, the more deeply they were able to look into the reality of matter, the further they seemed to be from simple and direct explanations which would prove true in all circumstances.

The doctors encountered even more baffling problems. The fine theories simply refused to work out in practice, possibly because they failed to account for the real world in which the patient had to be treated. Doctors with the widest horizon began to see that social reforms were as much a part of the struggle against infectious disease as the campaign against germs.

But how to enlist the co-operation of the business-men and convince them that for the well-being of the community they must help to raise the standard of living all round? At the best of times businessmen were individualists whose actions centred mainly round their own personal interests. Now, contrary to all expectations, the twentieth century was proving a time of intense difficulties for industrialists of all the advanced countries. How was it possible to talk of reforms and improvements to men struggling to defend their personal fortunes against the inroads made by recurring slumps and economic crises?

How far could medicine and health standards progress in the explosive chaos of two World Wars, occurring within the lifetime and experience of one generation? How far could science advance, stimulated as it was by the most intense drive in all history to conquer nature and bend it to the uses of men in bitter and total warfare? Even if the drive in society were towards destructive ends, medicine was a healing art, and what it gained from scientific achievements must be turned to a life-giving purpose.

All this the twentieth century is now witnessing, and it is not easy to stand back and decide what is significant for future generations in the many-sided activities of the scientists and doctors of the atomic age. Unlike the Red Queen in *Alice*, we are moving all the time, even when we seem to be at a standstill, but it is exciting and important to look round and try to find our course. We shall be better able to see what promise medicine holds for the future when we have taken the measure of the recent past and all the influences which have produced the medicine of today.

The Rise of Modern Empires

From Babylon onwards the methods of empire building varied only in the ways in which power was exerted by empire-builders over the people who were drawn within their orbit. At some periods the monopoly in empire was held by the one country which had advanced far beyond any other in technical achievement; at other times, there was a close rivalry between fairly equally-balanced powers, which rivalry generally ended in head-on collisions with disaster for all concerned, but sometimes in the release of new and creative forces.

During the Industrial Revolution, it seemed that Britain could never lose the advantage she had gained through her industrial strength. While other nations were striving to overtake her, Britain was away ahead staking her claim on the raw materials and the wealth of human labour existing in those parts of the world which by European standards were "backward".

However, the speed-up of modern times implied that other

expanding countries, principally Germany, would soon be engaged in similar adventures far from home.

This exploitation of other lands was, in fact, the only solution that industrial enterprise could find to a problem that was new in man's history. The working population could not afford to buy the total output of the machines; clearly, markets had to be found elsewhere. But other countries had the same idea, and competition for these markets became fierce; it was also essential for industrialists to obtain possession at the cheapest rate of as many sources as possible of the world's supply of raw material.

In the last twenty years of the nineteenth century, England, France and Germany added millions of square miles of "colonial" countries to their Empires, and many additional millions of people lost their racial independence and became subject races.

In these changing circumstances, a new problem emerged. The earlier "do-as-you-please" methods had given freedom to the small man to expand and develop at a reasonable pace. But these financial activities which involved many countries demanded some planning and control; the enterprise had become too ambitious for single-handed effort. Without destroying private ownership, some of the larger financial organisations formed monopolies and cartels, directing their greatly increased power against rival organisations; the incentive to this paradoxical planning amidst chaos was the ever-growing wealth that could be kept in the hands that controlled monopolies. Profit was for the small fry; super-profit was the target of the international financiers. To that end they re-organised and streamlined production; factories grew into co-operative giants engaging thousands of hands and producing more than enough for a nation's apparent requirements, with the highest rates of profit.

If the same methods had been applied to less profitable enterprises such as agriculture and to improving housing and living conditions, then the people and the doctors could have rejoiced; they would have been facing health problems linked with preventive, positive medicine, and leaving diseases of poverty far behind.

It could not be so, however, for one obstinate fact; capital was invested for profit; not for love, or pity, or even enlightened self-interest: the motive was profit, and the system had to be made to work to that end. All the subsequent events which affected the lives and welfare of the citizens of the Empire followed logically.

Financiers found that a higher rate of profit could be earned by investing capital in the backward countries rather than at home. So the coloured peoples, whose cultures and development had not directed them along the scientific path to imperial power, nevertheless found themselves making a contribution to the glories of empire. Like their white brothers in the Mother Country, they joined the modern army of wage earners, but at very much lower rates of pay. Like them they toiled in the mines and at the machines to aid the greater accumulation of capital.

Where the marvellous achievements of modern science could advance the cause of capital, no difficulty was found in transporting them into use in the colonies. So these primitive peoples learned to use and master the astonishing steam-driven railways and the powerful drills which wrenched the diamonds and the gold ore from the surrounding rock in which they had lain for long ages.

The major benefits of civilisation, however, were not exported for the use of those millions whose labour had contributed to their production. The Dark Continent of Africa (nine-tenths already embodied in one European Empire or another, by the opening of the twentieth century) remained innocent of any widespread use of electricity, mechanical aids for agriculture or other modern aids to prosperity and comfort; excepting where the white settlers found it necessary, for business or personal reasons, to improve the local amenities.

The medical services were equally crude; a thin façade, perhaps, would be constructed for immediate practical purposes, but the structure behind remained primitive. Yet these coloured peoples were being thrust, on their own ground, into a mode of life thousands of years away from their normal custom. It was a transition requiring the deepest brotherly sympathy and psychological insight: qualities in which it would not be profitable for industrialists to indulge.

The Clash of Titans

It had seemed at first that no other power could outpace the Great British Empire, but that did not discourage the other Empire builders. By the twentieth century, the world was already partitioned, with the Lion claiming the greatest portion; a claim that did not go un-challenged. Britain's achievements in industry and military might were closely paralleled by her nearest rival, Imperial Germany. The greater the power of the various monopolies and trusts, the greater the developing rivalries—and, the greater and the more disastrous the military clash when it inevitably came.

Medical theory and practice had always been affected by war, whose outcome is always settled over the broken and destroyed bodies of men, and in modern times, of women and children as well. The cataclysmic destruction of the two World Wars provided medicine with a vast field for exploration and invention. In addition, between the killings, two new civilisations arose, in Russia and in China; in these countries, medicine was violently shaken out of conventional channels and took an adventurous new turn towards social medicine.

Out of the clash of titanic powers, perhaps the greatest victory had been gained by the sciences, which in all advanced countries were enriched by the efforts they had been compelled to make in the cause of waging war. And when the titans were forced to withdraw from the general slaughter and took time to heal their wounds, medicine was able to absorb the knowledge wrested from a world agony, which could yet be turned to the salvation of man.

The Wonders of the Modern World

The nineteenth century had seen many astonishing changes in scientific knowledge and theory. After thousands of years of grop-ing, man had now made for himself tools capable of penetrating many mysteries. Yet, when he began to put them to practical use, it seemed that he was not at the end, but at the beginning of understanding.

Even the time-mellowed theories on the nature of the world and of life had to change when experience became richer, and in some ways, more contradictory. The true scientist and medical man of the twentieth century approached his studies with a proper humility and a knowledge of his own limitations, and yet with a boldness and breadth of view that made him a worthy heir to the best traditions of the past.

As ever, the searchlight of enquiry was turned on the central figure of man himself. Once, it had been the tentative surface examination, with only a partial sanction from a disapproving society; then, after centuries, the anatomy of man had been explored; but the knowledge that was gained could only partly satisfy the many queries that came to the mind of the intelligent investigator. What happened inside the living body? That was the question, above all others, that demanded an answer. It seemed that it could never be answered; and then came the invention of the microscope, and man plus machine moved into a new world of discovery. The invention at the end of the nineteenth century of the X-ray machine at last made it possible to reveal man to himself. At first this unique method of photographing the interior of a dense body was used in the simplest medical detection. Such irritants as stones in the kidney and bladder could be located, so giving greater aid to the surgeon.

But this discovery of X-rays had as many brilliant facets as a diamond. Eager and restless to test its powers, medical men were soon looking with new vision at the different injuries and diseases that could harm man. As well as tap the exterior walls of the chest and listen hopefully as though behind closed doors, they could now see into it as through a window. And then, during the First World War, the X-ray eye was employed to search out the odd pieces of metal and shrapnel which had struck at random but had failed to kill.

But there is much more to man than his bare skeleton. What happened inside the thirty feet of intestines which could, when irritated, cause so much trouble and even ill-temper in the owner? Other organs, such as the gall bladder, the kidney, the urinary system and the heart had secrets which doctors were eager to uncover.

New techniques were found to widen the scope of the X-ray; special harmless dyes picked out the organ under examination; a stodgy meal of barium rendered the stomach visible under the X-ray.

The study of the body in sickness was urgent; there was a long-term interest, however, in watching the normal workings of the inner man—for example, the means by which the stomach expressed its hunger, and how it did its daily grind in digesting food. The X-rays could give a tantalising shadow-picture of these functions to the scientists peering through the gloom of the darkened examination room.

Technical achievements, however, were almost keeping pace with the growing demand for more information. The art of the cinema had already shown a scientific bent when its facility to slow or speed up natural movements had been applied to processes of growth and action. Television added to this a bright chance of making the exposed X-ray film as clearly visible as the ordinary film. This technical advance means a revolutionary step for medicine; all the active members of the body may now come under the closest scrutiny; the swift, rhythmic movement of the heart may be slowed down for better observation without one second's inconvenience to its owner. A new and living chapter will be added to the great book of medical knowledge.

Electricity brings Light to Medicine

Medicine looked towards all the new technical wonders of the age for possible allies in the fight against disease. What were the chances of using electrical power in diagnosis or treatment? To the lay public it had already suggested itself (or had been suggested by cunning salesmen) as having some mysterious effect on the human body. The scientific approach, of course, was much more practical, and led to its application to delicate precision machines which could be used in medical tests. The electrical changes in the heart and brain could be recorded by the electro-cardiograph and the electro-encephalograph. What a wealth of knowledge they gave to the specialist. All the important actions of the heart, its beat, muscle-control, the speed and pressure of the circulation, could now be measured accurately in sickness and health.

The study of the electrical changes of the brain proved even more interesting. It was shown that every action had its corresponding electrical reaction; the machine made quite different recordings when man was asleep or awake, calm or excited; most important for the doctor, some diseases had clearly defined electrical patterns, as in epilepsy.

The further development of the microscope with the aid of electrical technique produced striking results. The common rate of magnification could now be increased up to 60,000 times, and the definition of the image was even sharper. Surprising new facts came to light. There, at last, for anyone to see, were the organisms whose existence had only been guessed; infinitely small as they were, they could now be measured and even compared with protein molecules, the very essence and substance of life.

The minute organisms were very much alive. Some of their activities were dangerous to health, but others were very helpful, such as the bodies which were used in the vaccine against smallpox, and the bacteriophage, which lived as parasites on some of the deadly germs.

No time was lost in bringing under the new super-powered microscope that fascinating structure, the cell. With the aid of cinematography, scientists were soon watching cells at work, carrying out the inmost mysteries of life, absorbing nourishment, removing waste products, dividing and renewing themselves. Nothing, it seemed, could remain hidden from the eye of the modern microscope; photographs were taken even of the genes contained within the nucleus of the cell, and carrying the very seeds of inheritance.

This approach was very different from the old methods of staining dead tissues with dyes, and then wondering how much of what one saw had been produced during life in the natural course of disease and how much in the laboratory. It was soon realised that it was more difficult in this than in any other science to reproduce conditions in the laboratory to coincide with what happened in the outside world; there was clearly a marked difference between the behaviour of living things as seen under the microscope, and as they really are in their natural environment.

The Chemistry of Living Matter

The fascinating study of the very structure of life really began in earnest at the end of the nineteenth century with the pioneer work of the physicists who were trying to reach the final analysis of inanimate matter. The atom was, after all, not the end: it had a nucleus with particles charged with electricity revolving around it. Matter was found to be held together not on a solid material basis, but in a dynamic balance with a controlled continuous process of movement. To those who, by training, were able to grasp the idea fully, this new reality was full of staggering and far-reaching implications. With imagination tingling, physicists searched for the proofs of the immense energy in the world around them.

Scientists had penetrated an invisible curtain; now they were going forward towards the control of infinite power and energy. Pierre and Marie Curie led the way when they discovered how to extract radium from pitch-blende, and revealed the form of energy, radio-activity, which radium was continually emitting as a result of atomic changes.

The new physics were applied to medical studies. The medical uses of radioactivity make a story of fascinating and promising adventures pursued by a team of experts—physicists, chemists and doctors. The actual treatment of cases is limited to certain forms of cancer and some allied diseases, but the range of research which is in progress is very wide; truly it is modern medicine in the making.

Doctors had long searched for more precise information on the action and distribution of chemicals in the body. How could one label an atom of a chemical such as iodine in such a way that its journey through the patient could be traced? The seemingly impossible was achieved through the knowledge of radioactivity.

Radioactive compounds of ordinary elements such as calcium, iodine and phosphorus can be manufactured, and when taken into the body the part they play in the chemical processes can be followed by the rays they emit. Soldiers of the atomic age and prospectors of uranium are familiar with the use of the Geiger-counter. The "click" of the loudspeaker and the movement of the needle on the scale indicate the presence of the element, whose progress through the body is being traced, as soon as the testing instrument approaches its location in the body. This is a valuable help in the recognition of thyroid disorders, in locating tumours of the brain, and in the treatment of thyroid, blood and other diseases.

At the same time, the X-rays that played such an important role in illuminating the inner recesses of the body, helped to shed light on the mysteries of the complicated molecules that make up the substance of the cells.

Just as a diamond, a crystal of carbon, or cut-glass sparkles when a beam of light passes through it and breaks up into many rays, so when a beam of X-rays is directed at a crystal such as common salt, the rays that emerge can be caught as a picture on a photographic film, where they make a recognisable pattern, which is determined by their speed and direction at the moment they are photographed. The pattern reflects the make-up of the crystal, and its structure can be discerned by measuring the directions and intensities of the rays as shown on the picture.

This type of new information concerning cells and molecules reveals the constant dynamic change that takes place in the structure and function of living matter. It is clear that within a matter of months, the tissues and organs of the body have an almost complete renewal of cells and substances without apparently themselves undergoing any change. It is this capacity to change in miniature and yet remain practically the same in general structure, which is one of the secrets of the ready adaptability of the body to its environment, particularly in counteracting adverse factors.

The Body at Work

Studies of the central nervous system had taught how the activities of the body were controlled and regulated by the nerves, spinal cord and brain. But at the beginning of the twentieth century another form of control was discovered, namely, the hormones, "the chemical messengers", secreted by the ductless glands and passing directly into the blood.

The action of hormones was studied in the now familiar scientific manner. Clinical observations were related to examinations of diseased glands and combined with experiments on animals. Individual glands were removed and the effects compared with the results of injecting chemical extracts of the gland. More opportunities for study were taken when patients had to have tumours or glands removed, and their condition was compared with that when hormones were injected.

Soon many disorders were traced to failures in the proper functioning of these glands: they included gigantism, dwarfism, diabetes and sexual precocity. The function of two of the ductless glands, the pineal and the thymus, is still not clear, although removal of the thymus gland appears to give some relief in an uncommon disease known as myasthenia gravis, a wasting of the muscles of the body.

Investigations made it clear that the ductless glands have a profound influence on growth, temperament, sexual development and the chemical changes in the body. Some hormonal secretions have special duties; for example, the adrenal glands pour adrenalin into the blood whenever there is an emergency which causes rage, fear or excitement, so that the body is prepared for the crisis.

The extracts of the glands are very helpful in medical treatment; not only in diseases such as diabetes, myxoedema and cretinism, which are caused by defects in secretion, but also in other apparently quite unrelated conditions. Adrenalin has proved beneficial in cases of asthma, pituitary extract for diabetes insipidus, and as a stimulant of the womb; recently oestrogens (hormones of the female sex-glands) have been found to prevent the spread and growth of cancer of the prostate; and to a lesser extent, both oestrogens and androgens (male sex hormones) have been helpful in preventing the spread of breast cancer. This latest knowledge points a new way forward in cancer research and raises profoundly interesting questions concerning the action of hormones in the general functioning of the body.

The study of hormones had arisen out of the examination of the changes in the structure of the ductless glands in the same way as diseases were related to changes in different organs. When the important role played by the secretions was recognised, the emphasis in study of diseases shifted from the disorders of the cells in specific organs to disorders of function in the ductless glands. At first the glands were studied separately, but it was soon found that they worked in concert to preserve the harmony of action of the different organs and parts of the body.

The latest extract, cortisone, derived from the adrenal glands and working in close association with the pituitary and other glands, has proved helpful in treating rheumatism and allergic disorders, and in strengthening the body's immunity to disease. This illustrates clearly that the ductless glands play an important part in adjusting the body to the environment, particularly in adapting it to conditions of stress caused by infection, injury, poison and other adverse conditions in the environment.

Food to Build the Body

People have always sought to satisfy their hunger, but the science of nutrition which achieved maturity in the twentieth century proved that it was not enough to satisfy hunger: quality as well as quantity was important.

Firstly, food has to supply the sugar and fats for producing the energy that all tissues and organs of the body use to keep alive and active; for example, energy must be supplied for the heart beating all the time, the chest moving regularly, and the stomach and intestines digesting food constantly. Secondly, food has to supply the material for the repair and growth of the body, and for replacements of worn-out tissues. Lastly, food helps in protecting the body from specific diseases and general ill-health.

There was already some knowledge of the elements in food that protected the body in certain disorders. Lind and Cook had led the way in the prevention of scurvy by adding fruit juice to the diet of sailors, so that the British sailor earned the nickname of "Limey" in the United States, because of the inclusion of limes in his food (now known to contain little Vitamin C in comparison with other fruits such as lemons, oranges and black currants).

In other lands, especially in the Dutch East Indies, there was a very common disease, beri-beri, which attacks the nerves, causing paralysis of the muscles and swelling of the feet. A young Dutch scientist who was sent to study the disease tried unsuccessfully for two years to find a germ which could be the cause. One day he noticed that chickens feeding from the waste food in the hospital grounds also suffered from the disease. He then found that the chickens who were fed on polished rice from the hospital developed beri-beri, but those who were fed on whole rice which had not been milled stayed healthy and did not develop the disease. The essential element in the food which prevented beri-beri was present in the husks of the rice and was removed with the polishings.

At the beginning of the twentieth century a new and great advance was made in elucidating the essential ingredients in food. An Englishman, Sir Frederick Gowland Hopkins, carried out experiments with rats and demonstrated that there were small quantities of vital substances in milk that were essential to growth. He separated two groups of rats: the first group he fed on fresh milk alone, and the second group on a mixed diet of fats, carbohydrates and proteins, together with all the minerals then known to be in milk. The second group stopped growing, their fur came out, their health gradually became worse and they died: the group that were fed only on fresh milk grew and thrived and were in the best of health. This experiment showed that there were substances in milk which were not present in the specially prepared food. These substances were named vitamins; and as the growth vitamin was the first to be discovered, it was named Vitamin A.

This discovery set the pace in the search for more vitamins, and within a few years three more were discovered and named: Vitamin B, for preventing beri-beri; C, for scurvy; and D, for rickets. Many more vitamins have since been discovered, each playing an important part in keeping the body healthy; the latest, discovered only a few years ago, Vitamin B12, has been effective in the treatment of pernicious anaemia.

This important study of nutrition was extended, with the discovery of vitamins, to a full analysis of the foods that protect the body and help in its growth. It was recognised that vitamins were essential not only to ward off particular disorders, but that, like hormones, they played their part in the general maintenance of good health, and in the body's defence against germs. A good diet was clearly necessary for adequate growth and health. This realisation profoundly influenced the development of agriculture and social relations generally.

Starvation was an ugly word with social as well as medical significance. Governments became interested when wartime experience revealed the deep-rooted consequences of widespread starvation. In the First World War, the defeat of Germany was due partly to the lowered resistance to disease and weakened morale due to malnutrition. In the Second World War, the British Government showed they had learned the lesson and included adequate feeding of the population in their defence measures. For the first time in history mothers and children were assured of the supply of vitamins and basic foods necessary for health and growth; the general population were protected from the dangers of short supplies by a rationing system. This far-sighted policy made a considerable contribution to victory.

Nevertheless, even in the modern, peacetime world, man's oldest enemy, hunger, still gains many a dreadful victory. "Women and

children first" might well be the slogan of such diseases as kwashio-
kor, only recently recognised by doctors as a disease of starvation
commonly found in early childhood in most tropical and sub-tropical
countries. The healthiest baby, when he is weaned, can be reduced
to a sick creature with mental deterioration, through lack of good
protein in the diet. The remedy is simple—milk. But many children
may yet suffer before adequate precautions are taken to protect them
from diseases of starvation.

Mind and Brain

The use of psychological methods of treatment was nothing new,
even to witch-doctors; but it was not until the nineteenth century
that it became a subject for scientific discussion.

Towards the end of the nineteenth century, the great French neuro-
logist, Charcot, employed hypnotism to cure a patient. His pupil,
Freud, analysed the methods which in the past had been associated
with much cheap sensationalism. Freud discerned an effect of hypnosis which led him to original and important conclusions. The
patient under treatment frequently recollected unpleasant or painful
experiences which he forgot when recovered from his state of hypnosis. The symptoms of ill-health, Freud reasoned, could be accounted
for by disturbed emotions resulting from these repressed memories
which, buried in the unconscious, were constantly trying to reach the
level of consciousness. The emotional conflict between the conscious
and the unconscious produced a troubled mind which could cause
sickness or an unbalanced personality.

The priest-healers of the Temples of Aesculapius had encouraged
mental "catharsis", the purging of the soul, and were skilled in the
art of the miracle-monger; the Freudian doctors introduced the purging of the unconscious and the powerful weapon of "suggestion",
to make the patient aware of the repressed experiences and so avoid
anxiety and emotional disorders. The patient was encouraged to talk
freely, expressing all that passed through his mind, whether relevant
or irrelevant, to the sympathetic and understanding psycho-analyst,
thus bringing unpleasant experiences to the surface of consciousness.
Freudians placed a special emphasis on the powerful instinctive drives,
particularly those of sexual origin. They concentrated on the "stream

of thought" and apparently meaningless details of dreams which, they suggested, if correctly interpreted, would reveal the cause of the disturbance. Unfortunately, the interpretations could vary considerably according to which psychiatrist was consulted.

The theory of the unconscious and the recognition of the effects of emotional disturbance on bodily functions was an important contribution to medical science, and helped to relieve the distress of many patients with neurotic symptoms. Thousands of patients gained benefits from the new teaching, which introduced a matter-of-fact and scientific attitude to people suffering from mental troubles, and placed them on the same level as those suffering from other forms of ill health. Nevertheless, because there is still no agreed scientific basis of diagnosis or test of cure, schools of psychoanalysis are founded on different theories and principles, so adding confusion to a difficult science, and leaving important questions unsettled.

Too much emphasis on the significance of inherited factors and repressed experiences of childhood discourages an optimistic approach to effective preventive measures. Psychiatrists generally see their patients as victims of a conflict between their conscious and unconscious, with society playing a major part in repressing man's basic instincts and urges. But many people are unhappy and insecure because of conflicts not in themselves but in society. Man, however, has always had to learn to live as part of a larger unit; he can gain immeasurably from a social organisation designed to strengthen human dignity and self-respect. Psychiatry will win substantial victories in the prevention of mental ill-health when it recognises that man cannot be separated from the effects of his social structure and environment.

Another approach to emotional and mental disturbances was made by the Russian physiologist, Pavlov. The controlling system of all the activities of the body was known to be the central nervous system, with the brain as the supreme functioning organ. Pavlov extended our knowledge of the functioning of the brain and in the process took important steps towards bridging the gap between body and mind and relating their activities to the environment. His careful and original research into the action of the brain and the basis of conditioned reflexes helped to explain normal and pathological mental activities.

Animals respond to changes in their environment by reflex actions which usually occur automatically. Many of these reflexes are inborn, common to all members of the species; others are conditioned, brought into existence by experience: they can inhibit as well as stimulate action.

The reflexes are associated with physical activities in the brain. Pavlov made a special study of the way in which they were established, and how they can be developed and retarded. Many of his experiments were made on dogs; he was able to induce mental irritability and strain, corresponding to the human "nervous breakdown", in animals confronted with problems beyond their capacity to solve, and especially if they were faced with a difficult choice between two paths of action.

Like animals, human beings acquire conditioned reflexes through experience; the senses, muscles and tissues respond through external stimulation. In this way man learns to walk, to think, behave and act as a social being, communicating his thoughts through one of the most important of social functions, speech.

Physical methods also are used in treatment but are not based on the principles of either the Freudian or Pavlovian schools. Some success has been gained in treating general paralysis of the insane by inducing fever, and depression and schizophrenia by the modern methods of shock treatment and surgical operations on the brain. However, cures are often temporary and partial, and occasionally there are serious personality changes. A fundamental weakness is the failure to associate these methods with a theory of the functions of the brain and their disturbance in mental disorders.

Because of the great increase in nervous disorders among the population of the advanced countries, it is becoming increasingly important to provide effective preventive measures. The emphasis on the role of the environment encourages a more hopeful approach, because it is much easier to change adverse elements in the social environment than to alter heredity or obscure happenings in childhood. Helpful methods of treatment can also be devised for individual patients. Already Pavlov's followers have applied his theories to treatment in inducing prolonged sleep, maintained over a period of many days with short interruptions for meals, and advances have been made in promoting painless childbirth and in elucidating the fundamental causes of many disorders, including acute rheumatism.

However, the main contribution has been the defining of disease as an unfavourable change for the individual in his interaction with his environment, which includes not only physical and biological elements, but also social relations. Preventive medicine, therefore, with a healthy mind in a healthy body as its main aim, must study man in combination with his environment, and investigate disease, both mental and physical, as a disturbance of the whole being.

War Against Germs

The knowledge of germs and their life history opened a new front in the battle for health. Society no longer had to struggle in the dark against contagious diseases; public health workers could discover the particular germ responsible for the outbreak, trace the paths taken in the spread of the disease and kill the germs outside the body; for example, they could purify germ-laden water, remove dirt and dust, and destroy insects and vermin carrying the germs of disease.

These modern methods produced results strikingly successful in comparison with past efforts, and hopes rose that soon infections and other diseases would come under control simply by finding the germ and destroying it, or by artificially strengthening the immunity of people who came in contact with the danger. But this mechanical approach was doomed as always to be confounded by the complications of real life.

Apart from the difficulty of discovering the germs, there was the problem of natural immunity and of germ-carriers, by no means simple matters to investigate.

Even today the germs causing the common cold, German measles, gastro-enteritis of infancy and others have not been discovered, and although the germs of poliomyelitis and other diseases are known, the route of infection has not been traced. Germs causing the common cold and measles cannot easily be transmitted to animals, and a searching investigation is not as yet possible; again, many viruses have been discovered causing influenza, so it is difficult to find a vaccine to give effective protection.

The problem of germ-carriers has presented equal difficulties. As far back as the Middle Ages it was recognised that the infected patient should be isolated; and this was a most important link in the chain of prevention of epidemics, but modern knowledge has shown that healthy people can carry the virulent germ and unwittingly spread it to those who are susceptible. How is it possible to find and isolate all the carriers in a large and changing population? Also, some people have the disorder in such a mild form that it is not diagnosed, and they, too, can unknowingly spread the germs.

Doctors soon came face to face with a related problem. At first they had assumed that an invasion of the body by a large number of virulent germs automatically resulted in an attack of the disease. Once again the mechanical approach proved inexact: some people developed the disease but others did not. Why was this? The conception of the body as a passive agent had to be re-adjusted. The recognition that the body could show active resistance to germs led to speculation and experiment with the process of immunity.

Jenner and Pasteur had covered new ground with their work on vaccination and inoculation, and their example was followed, with important results. It was found possible to stimulate the body to its own defence by injecting weakened cultures of the germs, or to protect it by giving ready-made antitoxins produced by animals such as the horse. Diphtheria antitoxin and immunisation are still the most important examples of this form of defence, and tetanus antitoxin has proved most valuable in preventing tetanus as a complication of road and farm accidents, and war wounds. Typhoid vaccine also saved the lives of many soldiers in the First World War in contrast with the South African War when the typhoid germs were more deadly than the bullets of the enemy. Since these encouraging beginnings, other important vaccines have been discovered, against plague, cholera, yellow fever, whooping cough, and the well-known B.C.G. against tuberculosis.

Nevertheless, the optimistic expectation that effective vaccines could be produced as soon as the germ was known was shown to be unrealistic; the greatest disappointment was the failure of tuberculin for treating tuberculosis.

One great drawback in this work was the fact that there was no scientific theory to guide action. The problems of the battle between the toxins of germs and the antitoxins of the body produced some ingenious suggestions, mostly unfounded. A well-known example was Metchnikoff's theory of killing germs by drinking milk containing lactic acid (yoghourt).

The main failure in forming a coherent view of germs and disease arose out of the failure to see disease as a changing process affecting man and his environment; the study of specific germs and the defence of the individual apart from his conditions of life could only touch part of the problem. It was also necessary to learn more about prevention and the building up of immunity by creating a favourable environment; but although this aspect was often ignored, the germ theory in general advanced preventive medicine by encouraging sanitary reforms and improvements in hygiene.

The new technique of dealing with disease by immunisation was not for long the medical wonder of the twentieth century. Ehrlich, who had laid the foundation for immunisation, discovered during his laboratory work that dyestuffs which stained germs in the test-tube could also kill them. His imagination was captured. If only he could find a drug which would seek out and kill germs in the body without damaging the tissue. From then onwards, Ehrlich devoted his life to the search for his "magic bullet". Quinine had proved a natural agent against malaria; there must be others, Ehrlich reasoned. He finally discovered the arsenic compounds, and by continually modifying the formula which he injected into mice, he produced some which killed specific germs without harming the body, including the famous "606" which, after 606 experiments, yielded the compound which was effective in sleeping sickness, syphilis and yaws.

These brilliant researches opened the splendid era of chemotherapy; incidentally, Ehrlich made an interesting observation during his work; in experimenting with parasites of sleeping sickness, he noticed that if he introduced doses of his drugs too small to remove the parasites quickly and effectively from the body, a new form of the germ developed, resistant to the drug.

The discovery of "606" held the place of honour among outstanding achievements in chemotherapy for the next twenty-five years. In 1935, the sulphonamides were manufactured, and they were developed into a wide range of effective drugs for many diseases, including pneumonia, gonorrhoea, cerebrospinal meningitis, scarlet fever, puerperal fever and dysentery. These drugs did not damage the living tissues, and seemed to be almost miraculous in their action; but as Ehrlich had seen, the battle of the germs was not to be one-sided, and new forms of drug-resistant germs soon appeared.

Then the struggle against germs was unexpectedly reinforced. In the late nineteen-twenties Alexander Fleming had made an interesting discovery. A spore of fungus was accidentally blown on to a bacteriological plate, and the bacteria surrounding the growth of the fungus were killed. Fleming did not do the usual thing and throw away the spoiled plate. With the unfailing curiosity of the true scientist, he investigated the reason for this effect and so discovered the germ-killing powers of penicillin, the product of the fungus. The potentialities of this discovery were not acted upon until the urgent needs of the Second World War spurred scientists all over the world to fresh activity. Large-scale production of penicillin was started in the United States, and it was soon found invaluable in solving many of the problems of infection common in war. Peacetime found even wider uses for this new "miracle" drug, which was less toxic than the sulphonamides and in some diseases even more effective; better still, penicillin could deal with many infections where, as in syphilis, the sulphonamides were ineffective. In some diseases where penicillin had no effect, such as typhoid, whooping cough and tuberculosis, other similar germ-killers like chlormycetin and streptomycin were soon produced.

Once again the old hope revived. Surely all that was now required was to find a sufficient number of drugs or antibiotics to deal with all germs? The answer came only too readily from nature; bacteriologists and physicians were not long in encountering new forms of the old germs, now resistant to penicillin and the other antibiotics; in fact, if the dose was too small, the drug-resistant germs flourished and grew on the challenge.

Now it seems that a race without end has started between the chemotherapists and the germs. At first the scientists were out to defeat the germs; now they must counteract the growth of drug-resistant strains of the germs; already they have speculated uneasily what would have been the position if the antibiotics had not been

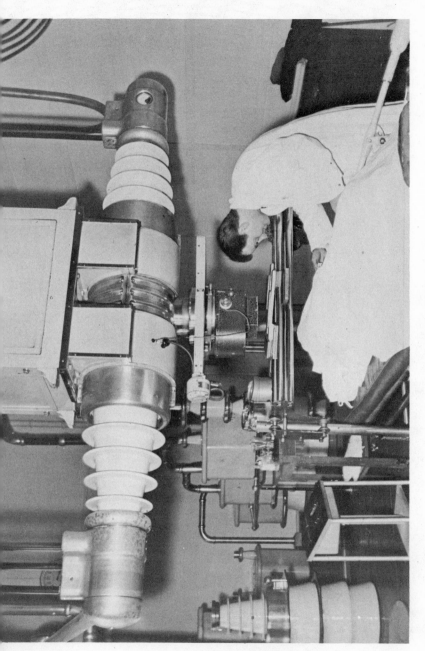

Modern medical machinery.

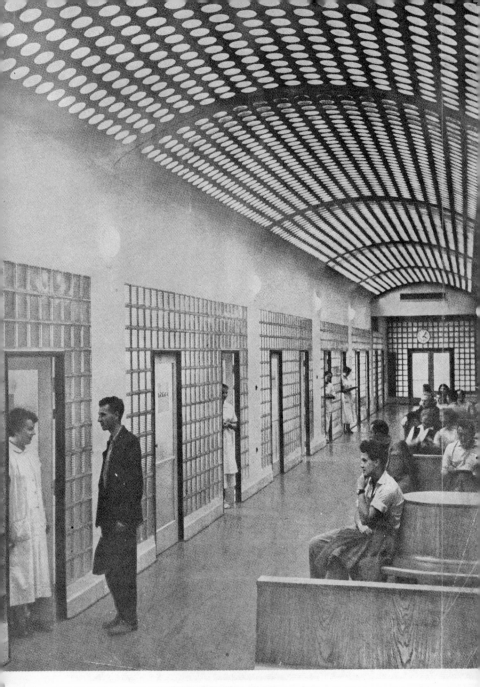

Health centre in Prague.

discovered to deal with the germs which by now would have developed resistant strains to the sulphonamides.

The science of chemotherapy has added valuable weapons to our
armaments in the battle against the germ, but without a coherent
theory there can be no guide to future action.

During the Second World War there were striking increases in
infectious diseases in countries which were occupied or under severe
attack; despite modern knowledge and treatment, it was clear that
infection spread in conditions which led to overcrowding and dis-
rupted sanitation; and in particular, malnutrition lowered resistance
and made people ready victims to disease. The most convincing proof
of the effect of bad conditions was the sudden rise in the death rate
of infants in the affected countries; as conditions improved, so the
amount of disease fell.

Similar comparisons have been made of the health of people living
in backward and advanced countries, or between groups living in
different circumstances in the same area. The findings consistently
support what most people know from their own experience and
observation—that it is healthier to live in an advanced country with
the amenities of good sanitation and modern public health protection, and healthier still to live in such countries in the best conditions
which are available, and which, unfortunately, are still enjoyed by
only a minority of the population. It should not be necessary to state
what appears self-evident—the best prevention against ill-health is to
build up the standards of living.

Tropical Diseases and the Colonies

The people in the colonies had greater health problems than those
in the temperate areas. In addition to the diseases prevalent in the
rest of the world, including typhoid, malaria, dysentery and tuberculosis, they suffered from those peculiar to tropical areas such as
yellow fever, sleeping sickness, and many diseases spread by insects
and pests which thrive in tropical conditions.

Most native peoples had low standards of living and poor resistance to infection; they succumbed in thousands to disease; the vulnerable infants in particular were wiped out by virulent attacks. They
did not benefit from the civilised amenities which provided pure

water, efficient drainage and better sanitation. They battled with disease, famine and drought, although not with the dangers and discomforts which were the common lot of the workers in the Industrial Revolution, who were forced to live crowded together in back-to-back houses in narrow streets, and to spend their days working in slum factories. However, industrialisation came to some areas of the colonies, bringing the same unhealthy conditions as in the mother countries. Tuberculosis, dysentery and malaria advanced against their weakened victims, and caused a doubled death rate in the newly developed colonies.

Nevertheless, some attention had to be paid by the colonisers to the conquest of tropical disease, otherwise no headway could be made in the important tasks of construction. Neither settlers nor natives could survive at this rate in zones teeming with deadly germs. The story of the Panama Canal neatly illustrates how diseases had to be conquered before progress could be made.

Empire-building had always been retarded by the commonplace affliction of malaria. This disease played a part in the decline and fall of the Roman Empire; and through the centuries it has plagued mankind; but it was not until the end of the nineteenth century that the parasite of malaria was first seen in the cells of the blood. In the same year work was begun on the important project of the Panama Canal, which was essential for the expansion of trade and navigation. For eight gruelling years, workers laboured in the tropical heat, thousands succumbing each year to malaria and other parasitic diseases. More than engineering and technical ability were required to carry out this ambitious scheme; in the face of failure to protect the health of the workers, the plan had to be abandoned.

Here was indeed a challenge to modern medicine, yet for twenty years it was not seriously taken up. It had long been observed that marshes, mosquitoes and malaria were connected; finally, the search for the parasite began in earnest. For two years of hard, unremitting work, the bodies of thousands of mosquitos were studied; and then, the reward of patience. The parasite was tracked down in the lining cells of the stomach of a certain species of mosquito; soon the whole picture was clear: how the parasite linked mosquito and man in completing its full life-cycle. The evidence was conclusive: men who were kept in a mosquito-proof hut in a malarial district did not contract the disease; others in a non-malarial district could be given the disease if they were bitten by mosquitoes that had fed on a patient with malaria. The answer to a centuries-old problem was clear: destroy adult mosquitoes and kill their larvae bred in swamps and marshes.

Fortified by this advance, a new start was made on the partly-completed and long rusted construction of the Panama Canal. President Theodore Roosevelt provided moral and financial backing; and this time a determined attack was made to control the breeding places of the mosquito, drain the swamps, and use chemicals in oil to suffocate and kill the larvae and the young growing mosquitos. The workers' resistance to disease was also raised by providing better sanitary conditions, doubling their wages and improving their diet. The Canal was triumphantly finished within ten years, with the saving of 70,000 lives and a sum of money ten times the cost of the preventive measures.

It is depressing to record that with this striking example before us, 100 million Indians will be stricken with malaria this year, of whom about two million will die; the economic loss is great and can be calculated; the loss to the well-being of the Indian people and the rest of the world cannot be measured.

Another brilliant page in the history of the medical conquest of malaria was written during World War II.

In 1942, Japan seized the main sources of the supply of quinine and derris root; quinine was the drug used to strengthen man's resistance to the disease and to kill the parasites in the blood, and derris root was used in manufacturing the chemical which killed mosquitoes. Substitutes had to be found immediately if the campaigns in the Far East were not to fail by men perishing in a greater number from parasites than from bullets.

Chemists in every country were pressed into the search, with adequate facilities for research, regardless of cost. Many anti-malarial drugs were discovered, some equalling, and others such as the British product paludrine, even more effective than quinine. Malaria menaced both sides impartially. Germany could not rely on help from her distant ally, Japan; and in her own highly-developed chemical industry she soon produced one of the best substitutes for quinine, chloroquine;

but in the German rout in North Africa chloroquine became a "prisoner of war". Under research, the drug soon revealed the secret of its manufacture and proved of great value in the campaign against malaria.

The war also gave an opportunity for a chemical discovered many years before to show its potentialities. D.D.T., now a household word, was found to be man's greatest ally against pests and vermin, including the mosquito. It was soon enlisted against the germ-carrying insects which spread malaria, yellow fever and typhus among the troops and the civilian population.

The opportunity came for a dramatic demonstration of its power. Naples in 1944 was a war-stricken city. At the cost of terrible destruction, the enemy had been driven out; in the shambles of the liberated city, the louse took over. Water supplies had been destroyed; there was little soap; dirt and poverty abounded. From one crowded living-place to another the vermin spread the parasite, and within a few days a typhus epidemic was raging. Hospitals were filled with the sick and the dying; cemetery-gates were never closed. The city was put out of bounds for the troops, but it could not remain an obstacle in the path of the advancing allies. Then D.D.T. was brought into action; the citizens queued hour after hour to be deloused by the simple application of the powder; the sick and the feeble were visited in their homes. Operation D.D.T. won the day and the louse retreated ignominiously. And history had been made: for the first time in the long struggle, man had controlled and ended an epidemic effectively and swiftly.

D.D.T. is a very recent achievement; previously, medicine found other ways to overcome epidemic fevers which were hindering the general progress of the nineteenth and twentieth century. At the same time as the mystery of malaria was being solved, efforts were being made to conquer yellow fever.

Along the eastern shores of North America where the greatest centres of industry were thriving, in Boston, Baltimore and New York, yellow fever ravaged the population; in Europe, Spain, Portugal and Italy also suffered greatly. At the end of the nineteenth century Madrid had a severe epidemic. In Sierra Leone one in every three white people died of yellow fever, every year. How could the work of colonisation prosper, with such destructive forces always threatening to cut down essential manpower?

Some attempt at control was made in an epidemic which broke out in Cuba, but the old tried methods of disinfection and isolation failed to arrest it. Clearly, the time had come for drastic action, and a medical committee was appointed with instructions to find at all costs the origin of the disease. Since the mosquito was the suspected cause of its spread, peacetime heroes had to be found who would volunteer for experiments. The doctors soon found soldiers prepared to risk their lives for an enduring cause. One volunteer was bitten by an infected mosquito and developed the disease; fortunately he recovered; another, accidently bitten, died after a few days' illness. This was convincing proof, but scientists must be thorough. Did the germ attack in any other way? Other volunteers shut themselves up in mosquito-proof huts; they dressed themselves in the soiled night-clothes of patients dying or already dead from yellow fever; they slept in the hot airless room on the very mattresses on which the sick people had lain—and they remained healthy and free from infection. The mosquito was the only culprit. The American sanitary department knew now where to direct their fire: yellow fever patients were carefully screened from mosquitoes, which were destroyed wherever they could be found. For the first time in 150 years, Havana was freed from the infection. The work of civilisation could push onwards with less interference from natural enemies.

But there was more yet to be learnt about fighting the yellow fever parasite. A new epidemic broke out in Peru, and nature was brought in this time on the side of man. Tiny fish called "millions" fed on the larvae of the mosquito, and these were planted to breed in ponds, tanks, reservoirs and rivers in infected areas where they effectively disposed of innumerable potential criminals, and greatly aided medicine in the control of yellow fever and malaria. Later D.D.T. joined the battle against yellow fever, which was as good as won.

One success was followed by another. At the beginning of the twentieth century the parasite of sleeping sickness was discovered in the blood of a patient and also in the body of the tsetse fly which was proved to be the carrier of the disease. The Indian Plague Commission proved that plague was communicated to man by the rat flea, and later both typhus and recurrent fever were shown to be carried by lice. Man could now wage a battle against these insects and rats, and after the discovery of the usefulness of D.D.T. in World War II, man thought he now had full power to end diseases carried by these pests. But just as the development of immunity through vaccines had its disappointments when the germs produced changes in their attack, so insects reacted to D.D.T. The balance in nature could not be manipulated so simply as men had hoped. Already resistant strains of insects have appeared, and also D.D.T. and its modifications have often destroyed useful insects that prey on the harmful ones. The effect of these chemical insecticides on animal and plant life have not been fully investigated; clearly, scientists have an important and interesting task ahead of them.

Nevertheless, much more can be done to eliminate these diseases with the knowledge we have. Man has the power in his hands to control the tropical diseases which until now have been the masters of humanity.

Today, one half of the human race, over 1,000 million human beings, still live in huts, cabins and slums in which it would be a disgrace to keep domestic animals; these millions suffer, if not from hunger, then certainly from malnutrition which saps their health and strength. Disease reaps a frightening and ghastly harvest: malaria attacks 700 million, and only one in 350 of these receives treatment; 200 million suffer from parasitical diseases; 100 million have trachoma causing impaired sight; there are about ten million lepers, and only three in every hundred receive treatment with the new drugs that can defeat the disease.

Yet, in the modern world, these conditions can be overcome in a reasonable time, given the determination and opportunity. For example, in the Soviet Republic of Uzbekistan, where under the old system all the evils of colonialism had ruled, malaria was completely eliminated within eight years. How was this achieved? The whole population was drawn into the struggle, with thousands of volunteers enlisting, dozens of anti-malarial stations set up, and teams of doctors and health workers carrying out mass health education. Large areas of marshland were sprayed from the air. The drive against malaria was carried forward on every front simultaneously. In this way, the people freed themselves from this disease. The success of this action has shown the way for an equally energetic drive against other tropical diseases such as Leishmaniasis and Kala-azar.

Man is no longer handcuffed and blindfolded in his fight with these worldwide diseases; he sees the cause and the weapons are in his hands. When this knowledge is put effectively into operation in every country, the entire health, wealth and happiness of mankind will rise in a magnificent response to his efforts.

The Art and Skill of Modern Surgery

Although the new life-saving techniques had been introduced into surgery by Lister some years earlier, an operation was still a hazardous procedure at the beginning of the twentieth century. A patient might be operated on in his own home by the light of a candle, with the anxious family expecting no better treatment, and relying mainly on their prayers for a successful result. There was no greater cause for optimism even in the hospitals: surgical cases were usually admitted too late, and patients were still prepared in a hasty and inadequate way for an operation performed in an atmosphere swarming with unsuspected germs.

Today, revolutionary changes have completely altered surgical technique. No longer is the patient admitted hurriedly the day before the operation and discharged in haste. Modern methods of diagnosis with X-rays and biochemical tests inform the surgeon of almost all the difficulties that he might meet on the operating table. The patient is prepared with harmless drugs so that an effective anaesthesia can protect him from nervous strain, shock and pain throughout the proceedings. The most modern methods of blood storage and transfusion can shield the patient from shock both before and after the operation; drugs relax the abdominal muscles and help the surgeon to see the area more clearly and to have wider scope for his delicate manipulations.

Until the twentieth century era of antisepsis, infected wounds were as dangerous to the patients as the disorder which required treatment. This fear is now banished, a thing of the past. The equipment and technique of the surgeon of today moves him far from his top-hatted, frock-coated predecessor a mere generation or two back. He no longer wears the same frock-coat for both post-mortems and operations, relying on carbolic sprays to kill germs brought into the theatre. Today, he wears a long white coat, mask and rubber gloves, and his protective clothing is somewhat reminiscent of the medieval physician; but the protection now is for the patient and not for the doctor. In some operating theatres, even the air is filtered to remove germs. Germ-killers can now be given to the patient before he enters the operating theatre, and the operation can be performed under the cover of a penicillin "umbrella"; the patient is thus doubly protected, and his body is ready to overcome stray germs that might penetrate the heavy guard.

The modern surgeon can operate on almost any part of the body. But the advances in surgery have not always been unmixed blessings; the relative ease with which many operations could be performed led to some speculative adventures of doubtful value. As Lord Moynihan, a famous surgeon, said, "We have made surgery safe for the patient, we must make the patient safe for surgery." He was making a sly comment on the tendency of specialists to operate for the beauty and technique of the operation, without fully considering whether it was really necessary or effective. He himself in leading the work of abdominal surgery influenced other less experienced surgeons to avoid many unnecessary abdominal explorations.

With their status rising ever higher in the medical profession, surgeons specialised more on particular organs and parts of the body, becoming skilled craftsmen in carrying out specific operations. The general direction of medicine and pathology encouraged this specialisation; and public esteem greatly enhanced the reputation of the masters of particular surgical operations, which was much to the advantage of the specialist who depended financially mainly on people who could afford to pay heavy fees.

However, the role of the individual star performer in surgery was not consistent with the wider scientific basis of modern medicine, greatly developed during the two World Wars, and especially in the second. Practice, particularly in the field of fractures, required a highly efficient functioning team of physicians, surgeons, pathologists and anaesthetists, each playing an important part in the common task. The great surgeon acting as a supreme individualist is becoming out-dated: the modern surgeon is taking his place as an important member of a team and he also works together with those who supervise the after-care and recovery of the patient.

Nevertheless, much of surgery is still focussed on individual organs, with no proper basis supporting the specialised forms of treatment; for instance, surgical treatment of gastric ulcers, gall-stones, kidney and bladder stones, does not remove the causes of these conditions. Criticism of this form of approach has become more emphatic recently, particularly in the method of dealing with cancer as an anatomical exercise, with no real understanding of the underlying causes and course of the disorder.

When the origin of the many ailments at present treated by surgery are disclosed by scientific medical research, steps can be taken to prevent these disorders or treat them medically, and surgery will no longer be necessary to make good avoidable damage. Surgery will be required for injuries and congenital deformities only; and even the latter may by that time be preventable. The great skill and finesse of modern surgeons will be employed in other ways in the practice of the art of healing.

Medicine in Modern Times

As with surgery, it took some time before the striking advances made by experimental research were absorbed into clinical medicine. At the beginning of the twentieth century, the physician was still very much the individual, relying on his five senses with some assistance from simple instruments such as the stethoscope and an old-fashioned ophthalmoscope, together with a few urine tests and examinations of blood. The doctor's main purpose was to diagnose the complaint and alleviate symptoms; he was little concerned with prevention, and his effective treatments extended no further than a few specific remedies such as iron for anaemia, quinine for malaria and mercury for syphilis. He did not disdain the classical tradition which included the use of purgatives, morphia and digitalis; and like the ancients, he relied mainly on the healing power of nature. The absence of scientific reasons for the use of many of his medicinal remedies led the more conscientious physician to admit to the inquisitive student, "I don't pretend to explain it, but I have seen it do good".

Gradually, however, the work of biochemists, radiologists and others, together with all the mechanical aids to diagnosis, became an essential part of the doctor's equipment. There was so much to know about so many disorders—too much for any one man to absorb. Hormones, vitamins and chemotherapy provided effective treatment in a number of diseases, including diabetes, pernicious anaemia, rickets, pneumonia, meningitis and venereal diseases. As with surgeons, physicians were tempted to specialise, and there emerged experts on diseases of the skin, lungs, stomach and brain, and for specific disorders such as diabetes.

Specialist attention was rarely directed to the commoner illnesses such as the common cold, influenza, rheumatism, bronchitis and minor gastric disorders, which overworked general practitioners have daily to deal with among their patients living and working in poor conditions. The experts often paid much valuable attention to rare and "interesting" conditions which enhanced their reputations. Although all aspects of medicine naturally call for study and treatment, and the study of even rare conditions can often throw light on the basic principles of medicine, there was a tendency to overlook social conditions, preventive measures and the commoner disorders. The effect of this restricted approach in clinical medicine was the failure of doctors to be guided by the concept of social medicine, which alone could lead to the development of sound new medical theories.

It was, after all, the era of the mathematician and the mechanical brain. Small wonder that the laboratory test and the statistical check dominated the methods of clinical medicine. Every day the scientists produced new ways of testing the functions of the body, parallel with the laboratory experiments on animals. Physicians who thought they had discovered a new treatment had to curb their enthusiasm until their clinical experience was subjected to a rigorous statistical control; it was felt that figures, being non-human, could not lie or encourage self-deception; in the past, too many worthless and even harmful "cures" had persisted from one generation of doctors to another, because they had never undergone a valid scientific test.

Medical opinion swung over to almost complete reliance on the laboratory and the guidance of the calculating machine, which was not constructed, however, to deal with the complex problem of the

interaction between the sick person and the social setting from which
he could not be abstracted.

There were some physicians who resisted this tendency to raise
totems to the modern gods of science. Sir Thomas Lewis, who added
considerably to our knowledge of heart disorders, fought the obsession that "useful discoveries are the prerogative of the laboratories";
and he and Sir William Osler reintroduced the bedside method of
instruction and research, and brought the methods of science to the
patient.

There was also criticism of the rigid way in which the results of
animal experiments were applied to man. Although much useful
knowledge had been gained about how the body worked, it had also
been found that different species of animals reacted quite differently
to many experiments. It was not only important to test the results
from one class of animal to another, but the final experiments had to
be made, if possible, on man himself. Modern students are fully
aware of this and frequently offer themselves as human guinea-pigs,
and a good many experiments are carried out, provided of course
they do not involve a serious risk.

However, the most important drawback to the value of laboratory
experiments with animals is that they do not live in socially organised
civilised communities as men do, and the factors in the environment
which affect health are not easily reproduced in the laboratory. This
is not unimportant, since it is fully recognised today that environment
deeply influences the evolution of many disorders.

Health as a Social Service

Two thousand years ago the Romans organised the first hospitals
in Europe; it was a humanitarian and important medical step but it
was also the beginning of a long struggle to make hospital services
adequate, and a well-balanced part of a complete health service. Two
thousand years would appear to be ample time for man to solve a
problem so necessary to his well-being, but the happy solution has
not yet been reached.

The English hospital tradition had for many centuries carried with
it the aura of charity, and those who could afford to pay employed
specialist attention and private nursing homes. The State had taken

the responsibility of providing hospitals for infectious diseases, a necessary precaution for the rest of the community. This was extended to serve the sick poor when no more could be done for them by those general practitioners who practised among poor communities for comparatively low fees; the sick and unemployed who could not afford even their low fees obtained treatment free from poor-law doctors after undergoing a test of their means. However, since the days of the Chartists and the early Co-operatives, the British people had learned the lesson that God helps those who help themselves, and they organised schemes of insurance through Trade Unions and Friendly Societies, which made provision for the misfortunes of ill health.

But while the population had separate services available to them according to their position and means, the advances in medicine and surgery stimulated changes progressing towards a unified service intended to benefit the whole community. Twentieth-century medical treatment involved the use of X-rays, biochemical examinations and other aids to diagnosis, elaborate operations, deep X-ray therapy, radium and other costly techniques. Not only the poor but also the middle class found these requirements quite beyond their means. Even the private nursing homes used by the specialists commanding high fees could not hope to include all this new equipment among their expensive amenities.

Scientific medicine had grown beyond the range of private enterprise; only the large hospitals could make the necessary provisions for scientific medical treatment; in the larger towns the new State hospitals began to cater for middle-class patients, and provide services equal to the voluntary or charitable hospitals. The challenge was taken up and the voluntary hospitals instituted private wards for paying patients as a means of meeting the higher costs of treatment. As a result there was some improvement in the general standards of all hospitals.

From the beginning of the century, efforts were made by organisations concerned with the welfare of the people to persuade Governments to co-ordinate and develop the health services available to the people.

In Britain we learned from the experience of the Boer War that without regular care a population will grow up physically defective, unfit to serve as soldiers, or even as peacetime citizens. Once regular school medical inspections were organised, it was found that Britain was painfully short of facilities for treating the majority of minor ailments or defects; eye, ear, nose and throat, and other clinics were established by the more progressive authorities, and open-air schools helped to bring the colour of health back to the pale faces of slum children.

The National Insurance Act of 1911 established a service of general practitioners for workers who contributed regularly through compulsory insurance; until the National Health Service Act of 1946, the wives and children were not included in the scheme, and many a pre-war general practitioner in this country can remember the mother with medical problems who never came to the surgery because of the few shillings she would have to pay.

At the beginning of the century, Britain lost 150 infants out of every 1,000 born, through lack of medical care and knowledge. The authorities organised important services which included health visitors and maternity and child welfare clinics; the health visitors went into the homes and helped mothers to care for their children, and doctors in the clinics supplemented this advice; at the same time mothers could obtain supplies of milk, milk foods and medicine.

The twentieth century will perhaps prove to be above all else the era of the mother and child. Ante-natal and post-natal clinics protect expectant and nursing mothers; a new, rational approach to childbirth is taught; Sairy Gamp is banished for ever, and all midwives are registered and are required to reach high standards to qualify.

People are health conscious; many a local and even national election is fought with promises for improvements in the health services as a prominent feature of the election programme. In the early days of the century, when labour and trade union representatives began to win seats in Parliament and Local Government, they played an important part in providing the health services which they knew from first-hand experience were so desperately needed by their constituents.

Yet many of these needs are still not dealt with in an organised way. Many people are still easy victims to a commercialism which does not hesitate to cash in on real or fancied fears of sick people by announcing special brands of some newly found drug. Millions of pounds and dollars are spent yearly on these and the older-style cure-alls. Large sums are invested by the proprietors in selling their patent medicines: on all sides insidious propaganda assails people: from out-size hoardings; in newspapers and magazines; and in America, on the radio and television; and neon lights flash the glad tidings day and night that "——'s" product will put you right. It is the modern method of sales-hypnosis and operates to the detriment of the public well-being. Not only do people spend on useless treatments money which would be better spent on wholesome food and other necessities; but precious time can be lost while the advertised remedies are being employed; modern scientific methods can be effective in the early stages of disorders, but frequently the disease has progressed too far before the proper help is sought.

The faith in patent medicines which has been raised to a constant state of fervour by the tremendous advertising campaign, also encourages the practice of non-orthodox practitioners, such as chiropracters, Christian Science and Faith Healers; in America these "doctors" represent one in five of those practising medicine. They seem as out of place in the twentieth century as was the witch-doctor in the classical period of Greek medicine.

People and Progress

The State and the Local Authorities had turned their attention to the health needs of the individual, but this does not imply that the battle to improve environmental conditions is over. In the advanced countries the sanitary reforms and improved water supply have brought an end to epidemics of cholera, typhoid and smallpox which spread like fire among tinder in the poor conditions bred from poverty. These dreaded diseases have been eliminated, but the slums and their evils remained. The number of deaths in different classes of the community can be neither manipulated nor misread. It was clear that the danger to health and life increases in relation to the bad living conditions of the people.

The figures were most eloquent during the grim period of 1930-5, when unemployment in Great Britain spread like an epidemic. In the derelict industrial areas malnutrition and overcrowding became the rule, as the people herded together in their increasing poverty and misery. The tables of sickness and death reflected the lowered standards in the wastage of infant lives and with a great rise in the numbers suffering from tuberculosis. Even in normal times, with all the efforts of the past fifty years of health and social workers, one-third of the population in America, Britain and Belgium are inadequately housed; one third have an income too small to provide the necessities for a healthy existence; and one out of every three school children, conscripts and adults is suffering from ill health or is disabled.

Man has had a struggle under normal peacetime conditions to create for himself a healthy and a happy life; but his most strenuous efforts have been continually undermined by outbreaks of war which have grown in destructive power until they threaten the modern world with complete catastrophe.

The wars of modern times have aggravated the poor standards of living of large sections of the population; as in Italy, they have caused the spread of epidemics by bomb-damage to the hard-won sanitary improvements; they have caused famine and starvation on a worldwide scale; in Europe alone more than 150 million people were left without shelter through incessant air raids; whole populations, vast armies, and thousands of prisoners of war, have had to be moved in haste and discomfort, with malaria and typhus and other infections moving with them—a cloud of disease over a wretched multitude of hungry and ill-tended people.

In war conditions the weakest fell first; in some countries half the infants died within the first year of their life; backward populations reverted to the worst periods of epidemics in history, and fell before the plague and other diseases as a result of the deterioration of their diet and mode of living and the disruption caused by battles. In parts of Europe the almost forgotten smallpox struck once more, and venereal diseases spread throughout the world.

The destructiveness of war continues long after the fighting ceases. Children and adults do not show physical scars to prove the mental and psychological damage they have sustained but they have suffered nevertheless, and sometimes have a life-long inability to readjust themselves to normal behaviour.

The intellectual life of the community is also interrupted in war-time, and many cultural treasures of the past are destroyed, and potentially creative artists and scientists are killed before they have been able to enrich the world by their work.

The standards of civilisation deteriorate in the chaos of a world conflict, and the sick, the aged and the weak are sacrificed by the reduced medical facilities which must be stretched over a far wider range of emergency cases. Humanity sowed the wind and reaped the whirlwind after the First World War, when no less than 700 million people were victims of an influenza epidemic which killed from fifteen to twenty million; history has no record of any greater devastation by epidemics, famines and wars.

It is true that science and medicine were stimulated to further advances by the needs of war, especially as money was made available for research; the teamwork of experts greatly strengthened medical practice, and new discoveries such as penicillin and D.D.T. were effectively adapted for peacetime uses.

The revulsion of the ordinary people against the senseless waste and destruction of war led them in peace to hope and plan for better and more constructive purposes; and out of this ambition the British people established the conception of the Welfare State with particular emphasis on the organisation of medicine so that the best service should be available to all who needed it, without financial consideration. Less thought was given however, to the need to protect health at work; the health laws for factories, mines and offices are old-fashioned and inadequate in comparison with the comprehensive provisions for medical care and attention in the home, community and school.

The new advances in medicine have helped to solve many long-standing problems but have brought into prominence others, mainly those associated with rheumatism and cancer, which afflict the growing numbers who are enabled by our better medical services to reach a ripe old age; other illnesses are connected with our modern civilisation, which in many ways places such strain on the individual that neuroses and mental disorders are a common problem; and we have yet to prove ourselves masters of the unspectacular but troublesome common cold, influenza and chronic bronchitis. The hazards of the

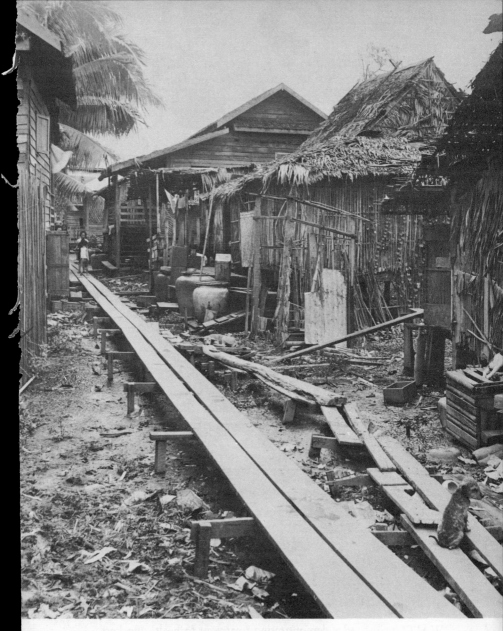

A typical colonial side-street.

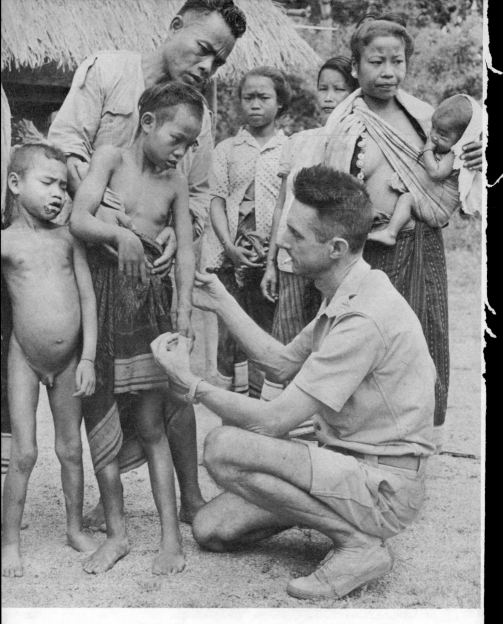

W.H.O. team leader demonstrating treatment to health workers.

jungle have been more than replaced by the dangers of the street-crossing; road accidents, and accidents in industry, have become a menace to the most active and productive of the population; the medical services are constantly employed in dealing with these preventable injuries.

A spectacular beginning has been made in the Soviet Union, where the creation of a new social order has also meant the development of a new, positive health service, concerned above all with the protection of the people at work, at recreation and at home. A comprehensive industrial medical service guards the worker at all stages of employment, and has at its command a whole network of holiday homes and sanatoria devoted to keeping people well and to the rehabilitation of the sick or injured. The care of the mother and child, the concern for the aged, and the general planning and expansion of health services with the enthusiasm of all sections of health workers are outstanding features of medicine in the Soviet Union. The emphasis placed on early detection of disorders and the generous provisions made for research speak of the new, positive approach towards health, which can well be summed up in the old adage, prevention is better than cure.

The great promise of twentieth-century medicine has yet to be fulfilled throughout the world in replacing the old, haphazard system by a truly scientific and comprehensive service available to all. As our knowledge is progressively applied to present practice, experience and wisdom will grow; this is a practical task which must be tackled by scientists, doctors, health workers and the people working as a united team. When this is achieved internationally, medicine will have reached the end of one epoch, and will be facing a new era of unexampled brilliance.

Chapter Ten

POSTSCRIPT

Looking Forward

THE story of man and his struggle for health up to the present time is after all only a beginning in comparison with the promise the future holds.

It would be pleasant to enjoy the luxury of looking forward, if only a short way ahead, and it may be an encouragement to those who see the difficulties rather than the rewards in man's centuries of effort.

Even today, although the incredible practices of witchcraft have been finally eliminated from modern medicine, the basic problems of real health-work have still to be dealt with.

The enlightened people of our time know what the true purpose of medicine should be. The First Constitution of the World Health Organisation expresses it clearly:

"Health is a state of complete physical, mental and social well-being and not merely the absence of disease or infirmity."

This also affirms that "the enjoyment of the highest attainable standard of health is one of the fundamental rights of every human being without distinction of race, religion, political belief, economic or social condition".

We know, too, that peace and security cannot fully be attained without also establishing sound health for everyone; and for success in this aim, the vast differences existing today between one country and another must be dealt with.

This constitutes the problem that must be solved in order to create the well-being of the people of the future. In that future, the generations of healthy, happy people will find it difficult to picture us, always apparently sick from some ailment or injury, beginning to feel old at sixty; worshipping in others, such as film stars or football players, the physical beauty and fitness of which the majority are deprived.

The results of many investigations reveal the physical and mental ill health of the world of the nineteen-fifties. Our people are both profoundly clever and profoundly confused. In our cleverness we have learnt how to release the energy of the atom, which in the future will be the material basis of prosperity, leisure and freedom; yet today it is a source of terror, a weapon of destruction more powerful than has ever before been devised. The great cloud of the exploded hydrogen bomb hangs over the world threatening complete annihilation. Is it for this that man has struggled out of the jungle and the cave, overcoming so many natural obstacles until he has become the acknowledged master of the world? Can we not learn to master and discipline ourselves and our enormous ingenuity? Many people in our days must feel downcast and cynical; for not only does an atomic war threaten every living being, but preventable sickness and disease are widespread, especially in what are called "the backward countries".

And what will amaze our descendants is that all the great wealth and resources of the "advanced countries" is expended on producing more and more arms and weapons of destruction, including methods of spreading germs.

It will indeed be difficult for the people of the future to understand this, for they will recognise only one enemy, disease, and will combine all their forces in a world-wide defence of man's valuable good health.

We can look forward to the future with hope, believing that our generation will succeed in preventing the dreadful catastrophe of world war; an important part should be played by the doctors and the scientists who in particular can understand the danger and the promise that faces mankind.

In the next fifty years, with the co-operation of the government and the people in every country, medicine will at last be able to turn full attention on its real function, the prevention of ill-health; and the first essential steps must be to carry into immediate practice the two principles laid down by our World Health Organisation.

Firstly, that "governments have a responsibility for the health of their peoples which can be fulfilled only by the provision of adequate health and social measures". This principle must become a law of every land, for the people and the doctors to keep continuously under review.

Secondly, that "unequal development in different countries in the promotion of health and control of disease, especially communicable disease, is a common danger". Future generations may smile at the apparent childishness of this comment; why state the obvious? But, since the days of belief in witchcraft, it has been only by painful experience that man learned many truths that later seemed self-evident. It will in fact be a tremendous undertaking, calling for the best efforts of men of all colours and nationalities, to remove the common danger to world health inherent in the poverty and degradation of many millions of our people, in lands like India, Africa and the Americas.

The medical profession of tomorrow will experience an exhilarating release of energy and enthusiasm when they and the people together tackle this problem of creating positive good health.

We know today how great the task will be. Almost everyone suffers at some time from one or more of the common ailments: measles, influenza, "colds", rheumatism, and the disorders caused by the strain of living in these chaotic times: high blood pressure, heart disease, and the many forms of mental unhappiness and disturbance. About ninety per cent. of all illness can be attributed to about five per cent. of known diseases. If doctors could save one in each hundred doomed to die of high blood pressure and bronchitis, immense benefit would be brought to humanity.

By tackling in earnest this simple proposition, the medical profession will find itself on the way to a complete revolution in practice and purpose. Since prevention becomes the main aim, the established method of studying diseases in their final forms will be reversed; and by concentrating on studies of health, doctors will learn how to rectify minor deviations before they develop into serious disorders.

It will be a revelation to medical men when they establish standards of normal health. Pessimism in our days pervades the very atmosphere of medicine; how lacking in cheerfulness our young doctors become, when in their training there is scarcely any mention of good health, and so much to say about illness and its treatment. The "specialist" of our days sees only the sick and diseased organ or bone; he is very skilled indeed, but somewhere amidst all the erudition the real person, the human being, often escapes notice.

Doctors will have to learn to look at the world with fresh vision. People vary in different countries and climates; they can deviate in many respects from the "ideal" of physical fitness, and yet not be ill; the highest standards of health of today can be tomorrow over-topped by new improvements in the general conditions in which people work and live. The work of promoting positive health cannot advance until doctors and specialists study the population with special reference to the work and life of the individuals in different communities.

These doctors will indeed be pioneers; there is so much to learn about the way people react physically and mentally to their environment. It will be clearly recognised that a patient does not wake up one day with a duodenal ulcer, or fully developed cancer or heart disease, or psychological injury. The task of medicine is to follow the processes through from the earliest beginnings, and to deal effectively with all possible aggravating causes.

Naturally the doctors will not act without the support of the government and the people, but already the common constructive purpose of all nations is making possible the united action which in future times will be accepted as simple good sense in all circumstances.

For today, when wars and economic disorder breed infections everywhere, the terrible disease of tuberculosis is being tackled seriously. A hundred years ago, a person who was told he had tuberculosis knew he had received a sentence of early death. But in the 1940's and '50's, a great campaign is being waged to educate people to recognise early symptoms and to accept treatment; doctors can offer every hope of cure. In the future, the other factors will be more vigorously dealt with: the overcrowding, poor feeding, and anxiety regarding family and work. How profoundly glad doctors and medical workers will feel, knowing that their skill and care will no longer be undone once the patient returns to his normal life.

As with tuberculosis, so with other diseases. Cancer, the name of which people once whispered with horror, is today being examined from every aspect, so that it can be recognised at the onset, and treated by a variety of means. Already we have learned that many chemical substances can produce cancer; a connection between cancer of the lung with tobacco smoking and pollution of the air has already been proved. Future generations will wonder how people were able to breathe at all in the smoky cities, dirt and dust in the air all round, and factories, machines and smoke-stacks producing still more. With growing understanding, however, doctors and populations will in time be as horrified by the pollution of the air as people became a generation ago at the thought of polluted water.

The problems of cancer, bronchitis and other diseases can be related to the problems of an unhealthy environment at work and at home; and along those lines medical research and practical action will unite to achieve the conquest of these ailments and the establishment of the clean and healthful cities of tomorrow.

The revolution in outlook and method will of course be accompanied by a complete change in the organisation of the medical services. In the world of tomorrow, no one will work alone. Men will give a new reality to the old saying, "United we stand, divided we fall". When, for example, the newly-qualified doctor commences his duties, he will join a team where with his colleagues he will work in the spacious and perfectly equipped rooms of the Health Centre; outside the medical team, there will be the local families whose health they serve; they too will be associated with the Centre in many activities, coming to lectures, spreading health education among others, helping with important health projects. And behind them they will have the firm support of the government, and world contacts with brother nations through the many branches of the World Health Organisation.

But this excellent organisation will have to be created out of what would seem by comparison to be chaos. With all the serious worldwide problems of ill health to deal with, doctors and reformers will develop the forms of co-operation that are essential to success.

The foundation stone of all aspects of medicine will be the recognition that man and his environment are inseparable. With the support of the government, the bad home conditions that breed disease will be firmly dealt with. New blocks of spacious flats and houses will be rapidly built as a priority health measure. Food and nutrition will be studied among all sections of the people, for doctors have known for many years that an adequate diet is the best way to strengthen the resistance of the body against disease.

The advanced countries have already demonstrated even during war-time that better feeding safeguarded the lives and health of mothers and children.

Once it is acknowledged that it is in the general interest to raise standards all over the world, the one-time "backward" countries will be rapidly industrialised, mainly by the efforts of their own peoples, but with the advice and help of the more advanced countries; however, all the bitter lessons of the nineteenth and twentieth centuries will be learned at last, and together with the introduction of factories and machines, there will come the supervision of living conditions, hours of work and rates of pay, and the liberal provision of modern health centres and hospitals, clinics and trained workers. The expense of providing these conditions will be amply repaid by the increase in production and the reduction in the cost to the country of ill and helpless citizens. By the end of the momentous twentieth century, the coloured peoples may well be freed at last from the horrors of diseases such as yaws, hookworm and bilharziasis; the abundant and creative output of these millions of people will prove how much was lost to past generations through the pitiful failure of medicine and society to 'put their house in order'.

The medical profession will leap from one victory to another. The triumphs over disease will lead the way to positive action to promote good health. All the conditions that might cause deterioration in world standards will be constantly under supervision. Since food is the basis of good health, science will be applied to food production on a world scale, with the co-operation of all countries. Pests, infestations and diseases that spoil quantities of food can be dealt with by every chemical and scientific means; vast new tracts of land can be cultivated and soil erosion controlled. The interests of the farming communities will be well cared for, and their special health requirements in particular; for sick farmers cannot farm.

Naturally, there will be planning on a world scale to see that food supplies are evenly distributed so that no person will ever again have to fear hunger. Humanity will feel a shock of relief and astonishment when it is found that once the ancient rivalries are removed, there really is no serious obstacle to world co-operation; in fact, people everywhere will greet the new life with growing enthusiasm, for it will not merely be given to them by a remote authority, but will be a life of their own creation.

In every land, medical specialists will be called in to apply new methods of promoting good health. They will become guardians of health, for example, by examining all processed foods before they are released, and by testing all new chemical and factory processes to make certain they can be operated with safety.

Imperceptibly, the revolution in medicine will come about, and with it the revolution in the health of all peoples. It has taken man millions of years to progress from the fear of witchcraft to the hope of world health; and from that first glimpse at the future it need take only a generation or two to reach the fulfilment of that hope: a world of healthy, happy people at peace.

INDEX

Due